TRAUMA CARE SYSTEMS

TRAUMA CARE SYSTEMS

Clinical, Financial, and Political Considerations

Editor

John G. West, M.D.
Clinical Instructor in Surgery
University of California
California College of Medicine
Irvine, California

Associate Editors

Alan B. Gazzaniga, M.D.
Professor of Surgery
University of California
California College of Medicine
Irvine, California

Director, Trauma Service
University of California,
Irvine Medical Center
Orange, California

Richard H. Cales, M.D.
Clinical Instructor in Medicine
University of California
California College of Medicine
Irvine, California

Clinical Instructor in
Emergency Medicine
University of Southern California
Los Angeles, California

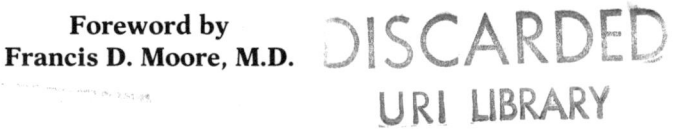

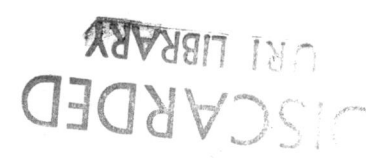

Foreword by
Francis D. Moore, M.D.

PRAEGER

PRAEGER SPECIAL STUDIES • PRAEGER SCIENTIFIC

Library of Congress Cataloging in Publication Data
Main entry under title:

Trauma care systems.

  Bibliography: p.
  Includes index.
  1. Wounds and injuries—Treatment—United States.
2. Wounds and injuries—Treatment—Economic aspects—
United States. 3. Wounds and injuries—Treatment—
Political aspects—United States. 4. Regional medical
programs—United States. I. West, John G. II. Gazzaniga,
Alan B. III. Cales, Richard H. [DNLM: 1. Emergency
medical services. 2. Wounds and injuries—Therapy. WO
700 T7756]
RD93.8.T7 1983   362.1'971'0973   83-11223
ISBN 0-03-063209-9

Published in 1983 by Praeger Publishers
CBS Educational and Professional Publishing
A Division of CBS, Inc.
521 Fifth Avenue, New York, New York 10175 U.S.A.

© 1983 by Praeger Publishers

All rights reserved

456789 052 98765432

Printed in the United States of America on acid-free paper.

To our families

Jan, Justin, and Matthew West

Shae, Catherine, David, Michael, and Andrea Gazzaniga

Carolyn, Christy, and Mark Cales

CONTRIBUTORS

Bruce M. Achauer, M.D.
Associate Professor of Surgery
Division of Plastic Surgery
University of California, Irvine
 Medical Center
Orange, California

Michael R. Antopol, M.D.
Colonel, Medical Corps,
 U.S. Army
Consultant in Surgery to the
 Surgeon General, U.S. Army

Richard H. Cales, M.D.
Clinical Instructor
Department of Internal
 Medicine
University of California
California College of Medicine
Irvine, California

Henry C. Cleveland, M.D.
Clinical Professor of Surgery
University of Colorado
Medical Director
Patient Care Services
St. Anthony's Hospital Systems
Denver, Colorado

Alasdair Conn, M.D.
Medical Director
Field Operations Program
Shock Trauma Unit
University of Maryland
Maryland Institute for
 Emergency Medical Services
 Systems
Baltimore, Maryland

Dan Dracon, M.D.
Emergency Services
St. Anthony's Hospital Systems
Denver, Colorado

John J. Fried
Editor, Editorial Pages
Independent Press Telegram
Long Beach, California

Alan B. Gazzaniga, M.D.
Professor of Surgery
University of California
California College of Medicine
Irvine, California

Frank R. Lewis, M.D.
Associate Professor of Surgery
University of California
San Francisco, California
Director, Emergency
  Department
San Francisco General Hospital
San Francisco, California

Charles R. McElroy, M.D.
Associate Clinical Professor of
  Medicine
University of California Medical
  Center
Los Angeles, California

Nina Merrill
Director, Life Flight of Southern
  California
Long Beach, California

Lawrence H. Pitts, M.D.
Associate Professor of
  Neurosurgery
University of California
San Francisco, California
Chief of Neurosurgery
San Francisco General Hospital
San Francisco, California

Bridget Simone, M.P.H.
Executive Director
Inland Counties Emergency
  Medical Authority
San Bernardino, California

C. Thomas Thompson, M.D.
Clinical Professor of Surgery
University of Oklahoma
Tulsa Medical College
Tulsa, Oklahoma
Chairman, Committee on
  Trauma
American College of Surgeons

Donald D. Trunkey, M.D.
Professor of Surgery
University of California
San Francisco, California
Chief of Surgery
San Francisco General Hospital
San Francisco, California

John G. West, M.D.
Clinical Instructor in Surgery
University of California
California College of Medicine
Irvine, California

Dennis A. Wheeler, M.D.
Medical Director
Inland Counties Emergency
  Medical Authority
San Bernardino, California
Director, Emergency
  Department
Pomona Valley Community
  Hospital
Pomona, California

Michael Williams, M.P.A.
President
EMS Systems Design
Irvine, California

FOREWORD

Over the years, the term "epidemiology" has called to mind such phenomena as ticks on rats bearing typhus to the people of Central Europe, a leaky sewer pipe drain causing typhoid in Northern Scotland, or mosquitoes in the swamps of Florida or Central America preventing the settlement of those regions. But now, the word "epidemiology" has gained a much broader meaning. We speak of the epidemiology of motor vehicle accidents and the epidemiology of trauma. By this is meant the distribution of vehicle accidents, the types of road construction that lead to accidents, the types of highway construction that deter accidents, and the detailed human engineering of motor vehicles so that lives may be saved and deformities may be avoided by design rather than by chance.

The epidemiology of trauma goes much further to understand the importance of the mechanism of injury. Not all burns arise from the same mechanism. Burns in children are more commonly scalds; burns in women more commonly are produced in the home, often in conjunction with alcohol; and for burns in men, an industrial site is common. Knowledge of the mechanism of injury will ultimately lead to prevention.

The term "epidemiology" has also come to include a look at the distribution of treatment modes. The epidemiology of heart transplantation, for example, was demonstrated by some early beginnings in the western part of the United States, a spectacular outburst in South Africa, and an abortive series of unsuccessful attempts in Texas, followed by the gradual and significant buildup of a successful experience in California. The epidemiology of cardiac surgery as a whole can similarly be traced to its places of origin and its gradual spread through the migration of experienced surgeons.

The epidemiology of the care of trauma is more complicated. One might naively conclude that treatment simply occurs where the accident happens and that the nearest hospital is the place of choice. It has always been evident to surgeons of the great wars that such a management, sorting, or triage of injury is disastrous. The nearest place might be the ideal spot for a minor injury or a simple fracture. But it might mean certain death if the injury is a closed head injury with a subdural or epidural hematoma. It spells certain death if the injury is secondary to a massive coronary occlusion whose recognition is apt to be overlooked at the nearest place. For injuries such as a ruptured spleen, liver, or small intestine, diagnostic methods that require an experienced hand or an experienced eye are essential.

This book by Dr. West, Dr. Gazzaniga, and Dr. Cales covers not only the epidemiology of trauma and its care, but it goes one step further, namely, it organizes the epidemiology of care.

To organize the distribution of this care one must think in terms of regions. The size of the region depends on its population and transport capability. It is influenced (although to a lesser extent) by the frequency of trauma in the area. It is also influenced by the distribution of various types of hospitals and by the identification of those hospitals that have highly experienced physicians and surgeons on duty or immediately available 24 hours a day. Most teenage alcohol vehicular accidents, often high speed, highly lethal, and involving serious head injury, occur in the early morning hours. There must be readily available emergency physicians, surgeons, anesthesiologists, etc.

This book fills a long perceived need. It does it better than any other. It is a privilege to have known the book in its formative stages, to have worked with its authors, and to feel a share in this new departure for the United States: organizing the epidemiology of trauma care to match the nature of the injury and its epidemiology.

FRANCIS D. MOORE, M.D.

PREFACE

Modern trauma care is a planned partnership between the community and the individual physician. It demands not only clinical management skills but also a coherent organization to bring those skills to the trauma victim. At a recent symposium, a group of nationally recognized trauma experts were invited to share their views on the development of a regional trauma system and how such a system would impact the medical community. This book includes selected topics from that symposium. We recognize that many areas in this country are now in the process of the actual development or implementation of such a regional trauma system. Therefore, it is essential to make this information available on a timely basis. To accomplish this, the subject matter presented will be taken for the most part directly from the talks as presented with only a limited amount of editing.

ACKNOWLEDGMENTS

The editors are pleased to have this opportunity to acknowledge many of the individuals who made this book possible. In particular, Dr. Leonard Berman's many valuable suggestions were instrumental in the development of the Orange County regional trauma system and ultimately led to the successful completion of this book. We are indebted to the many Orange County physicians who provided many precious hours of their time to perform the two Orange County trauma audits. The Orange County Board of Supervisors, the county health officer, Dr. Rex Ehling, and the county epidemiologist, Dr. Thomas Prendergast, have been instrumental in the design and maintenance of a high quality trauma system for Orange County.

The editors extend their appreciation to all the contributors for their numerous, thoughtful suggestions, and readiness to help. We wish to thank Janice Stewart for her many long hours spent in typing, organizing, and coordinating the materials necessary to complete this book. And finally we wish to thank Shirley Gower, the Executive Director of the Orange County Trauma Society, for many hours spent in organizing the symposium that led to the development of this book.

CONTENTS

CONTRIBUTORS		vii
FOREWORD		ix
Francis D. Moore, M.D.		
PREFACE		xi
ACKNOWLEDGMENTS		xiii
TRAUMA CARE: PAST, PRESENT, AND FUTURE		xvii
C. Thomas Thompson, M.D.		

PART I TRAUMA SYSTEMS DEVELOPMENT

1. PREDICTING THE COMMUNITY'S NEEDS: LOCAL SOLUTIONS TO LOCAL PROBLEMS — 5
   Donald D. Trunkey, M.D.
2. URBAN SYSTEMS OF TRAUMA CARE: THE BALTIMORE EXPERIENCE — 11
   Alasdair Conn, M.D.
3. RURAL SYSTEMS OF TRAUMA CARE: THE COLORADO EXPERIENCE — 14
   Henry C. Cleveland, M.D., Dan Dracon, M.D.
4. MEDICAL AUDIT OF TRAUMA SYSTEMS — 17
   Richard H. Cales, M.D.
5. THE TRAUMA CENTER DESIGNATION PROCESS — 27
   Michael Williams, M.P.A.
6. FINANCIAL CONSIDERATIONS — 37
   Michael Williams, M.P.A.
7. THE COMMUNITY HOSPITAL AS A TRAUMA CENTER — 55
   C. Thomas Thompson, M.D.
8. THE UNIVERSITY HOSPITAL AS A LEVEL I TRAUMA CENTER — 61
   Donald D. Trunkey, M.D.

PART II SPECIAL CLINICAL NEEDS IN TRAUMA SYSTEMS DEVELOPMENT

9. THE ROLE OF THE EMERGENCY PHYSICIAN — 73
   Charles R. McElroy, M.D.

10	PREHOSPITAL CARE: THE ROLE OF THE EMT-PARAMEDIC Frank R. Lewis, M.D.	77
11	MECHANISMS OF PREHOSPITAL IDENTIFICATION OF TRAUMA PATIENTS Dennis A. Wheeler, M.D., Bridget Simone, M.P.H.	86
12	PEDIATRIC TRAUMA: THE BALTIMORE EXPERIENCE Alasdair Conn, M.D.	91
13	AN AGGRESSIVE APPROACH TO THE NEUROLOGICALLY INJURED PATIENT Lawrence H. Pitts, M.D.	94
14	THE ORGANIZATION OF CARE FOR THE PATIENT WITH A SEVERED LIMB Bruce M. Achauer, M.D.	102
15	HELICOPTER TRANSPORT SYSTEMS Alasdair Conn, M.D., Nina Merrill	108
16	ADVANCES IN THE MILITARY MANAGEMENT OF MASS CASUALTIES Colonel Michael R. Antopol, M.D.	115
PART III	**A STRATEGY FOR IMPLEMENTATION OF A REGIONAL TRAUMA SYSTEM**	
17	DO TRAUMA SYSTEMS SAVE LIVES? John G. West, M.D., Alan B. Gazzaniga, M.D., Richard H. Cales, M.D.	129
18	METHODS OF EVALUATION OF TRAUMA CARE John G. West, M.D., Richard H. Cales, M.D.	141
19	OBSTRUCTIONS IN THE ROAD TO TRAUMA CARE: THE LOS ANGELES EXPERIENCE Charles R. McElroy, M.D.	152
20	INDEPENDENT PARTNERS: THE MEDIA AND MEDICINE John Fried	160
	EPILOGUE John G. West, M.D.	172
	INDEX	175

TRAUMA CARE: PAST, PRESENT, AND FUTURE
C. Thomas Thompson, M.D.

Patients with major injuries often tax the capabilities of hospitals and the skills and ingenuity of physicians entrusted with their care. The complexity of the problem is magnified by the multiplicity of patients. The differing needs of urban trauma patients in our crowded cities and the critically injured in rural America defy a uniform system. The economics of our entire medical system bears on our trauma epidemic. The cost to society in death and disability of our youth is a well-known statistic. The annual carnage on our highways surpasses that of the entire Vietnam War, and yet the public outcry seems strangely muffled.

It is perhaps easier to plan for medical care in wartime when there is a well-defined chain of command for the ultimate, planned trauma. The number of expected injuries is generally well-defined, and the echelons of care have been well-developed. On-scene treatment, transportation systems, and the utilization of protocols are excellent. These wartime skills for mass trauma, however, have not been generally applied to the civilian system. The independent nature of the American citizen has, perhaps, prevented the imposition of a military-type system in our private setting.

The drive toward regionalization of trauma care dates back to the mid-1960s. The landmark publication, "Accidental Death and Disability: The Neglected Disease of Modern Society,"* focused attention on this problem. Shortly thereafter, government agencies such

---

*National Academy of Science/National Research Council, 1964.

as the Department of Transportation and the Department of Health, Education and Welfare, as well as organized medicine, started to work on categorization of medical facilities. Numerous categorization schemes, variously called horizontal, vertical, and circular, were developed, and innumerable conferences and seminars led to city-, county-, and state-wide categorization plans. Most of these plans have simply gathered dust, however, for changes in patient flow have rarely occurred just because a plan has been written.

The Emergency Medical Services (EMS) Division of the Department of Health, Education and Welfare, under Dr. David Boyd, originally envisioned wall-to-wall EMS regions with designated trauma centers. The well-known 15 EMS components have provided a valuable tool in assessing the capabilities in trauma care by calling attention to many areas of deficiency. Historically, EMS has provided little money and even less power in its attempt to influence physicians and hospitals, resulting in compliance that has at best been spotty. Even the implication of imposing a governmental system has generally met with great resistance.

In 1976, a task force of the Committee on Trauma of the American College of Surgeons (ACS) published a document entitled, "Optimal Hospital Resources for Care of the Seriously Injured," which recommended that the seriously injured patient be given special consideration in the planning process. There was a clear call for hospitals to make a commitment to provide the facilities and personnel necessary to address the special problems of the seriously injured patient. In the 1979 revision of this document, the Committee on Trauma attempted to produce a pragmatic national guideline. The title reflected the change in emphasis, "Hospital Resources for Optimal Care of the Injured Patient."

Despite its obscure origin, the term "trauma center" has achieved wide acceptance in describing the development of hospitals specializing in trauma care. The American College of Surgeons' document does not use the term; instead, it emphasizes that the most significant single ingredient is commitment.

For the hospital, optimal care means provision of expensive personnel, equipment, and services. There must be a priority of access to sophisticated laboratory and radiological facilities as well as the operating suite and critical care units. The ultimate responsibility for commitment and quality of medical care rests with the board of trustees of individual hospitals.

For the medical staff, optimal care means a commitment to availability, education, and regular medical audits. The disruptive nature of trauma patients who arrive at unreasonable times, with unreasonable problems, and in frequently inconvenient numbers may cause the medical staff to opt out of a trauma commitment. The preemptive nature of the demands of the trauma patient for diagnostic services, operating suites, blood, and critical-care units may change the nature of an institution.

The linchpin of the entire system of trauma care is the surgeon—trauma is a surgical disease! It is for this reason that the American College of Surgeons has chosen to address this difficult problem. The quality of surgical leadership is of paramount importance in the development of a trauma program, for no successful trauma program can be developed without the express commitment of the surgical department. The demands in availability, surgical skills, judgment, and education are taxing. Any institution that wishes to make a commitment to excellence in trauma care must first assess its surgical staff.

The nature of the trauma patient requires a series of changing interfaces. The citizen on the scene, the emergency medical technician (EMT)-Paramedic, the emergency physician, the surgeon, the surgical specialist, the anesthesiologist, and the critical care team all have vital roles. If these roles are clearly defined, turf problems will be minimized and the continuum of care will be smooth. Ongoing medical audit of these roles is in the best interest of the patient.

The designation of trauma centers is essentially a protocol process that may be accomplished by a community or region willing to assess its capabilities. It requires leadership, statesmanship, and an earnest desire to improve patient care. The ACS Committee on Trauma responds to a broad range of requests for consultation on the development of trauma systems. The emphasis is on the voluntary commitment of the institution and the necessity for community involvement. The American College of Surgeons' effort is an attempt to provide a national standard for the measurement of an institution's capability to respond to the special demands of the severely injured patient. This can occur only if the community can articulate its needs in the trauma arena. The American College of Surgeons has no plan as such for the organization or regionalization of trauma care.

Where are we now in this trauma regionalization drive and where are we going? Centers of excellence for burn care, neonatal and perinatal care, and spinal cord injuries are available. The ambiguous nature of trauma and the difficulty of defining "serious injury" are a part of the problem. Certainly the patient with a broken leg should be treated by the physician of his choice at the hospital of his choice. The multiply injured patient in shock, however, may not have that option.

A few areas of the country have addressed some of the painful problems of regionalization. Where there is public awareness, good medical leadership, and organizational skills to marshal regional resources, the record is good. For most of the United States, however, citizens' apathy toward our national epidemic may preclude excellence in trauma care. The parochial attitude of hospitals, medical schools, and physicians continues to compound the problem. The economic factors relating to trauma care are staggering. The cost to society in dollars, as well as grief from death and disability, cannot be overemphasized. The ability of the private sector to meet the demands of escalating health-care costs is certainly in question. The private nonprofit hospital has a cloudy future according to most predictions, while there is considerable doubt that the for-profit hospitals will view trauma as a high priority. The effects of the injured indigent on the designation process are yet unknown. Certainly the economic factors cannot be left to chance in the planning process.

If the American citizen recognizes the nature of our trauma epidemic, then perhaps there will be a demand for centers providing excellent care for the severely injured. The daily litany of statistics devoted to our mayhem on the streets and highways, in our crowded cities, and in rural America perhaps benumbs us to the fact that these human beings are frequently our family and friends. The overwhelming problems of alcohol, drugs, gun control, and motorcycles seem political until they occur next door. The future of regionalization of trauma care with development of centers of excellence is entirely dependent upon our sense of priorities.

PART I
TRAUMA SYSTEMS DEVELOPMENT

Advances in trauma care are dependent on implementation of systems that provide state-of-the-art medical care for all trauma victims. In this section we will consider some of the methods utilized in the development of a long-range trauma plan based upon demonstrated need and available resources.

Introducing this section is a treatise by Dr. Donald D. Trunkey that addresses the issues of assessing needs in prehospital care, the number and location of trauma centers, and the services expected of a trauma center.

In Chapter Two, the complex medical needs and political realities of urban America are discussed by Alasdair Conn in the context of the Baltimore system where resources abound and competition for patients is intense. In stark contrast is the experience of Drs. Henry C. Cleveland and Dan Dracon, who discuss in Chapter Three the problems of scarce resources, low volumes, and long transports encountered in the rural west.

The next three chapters are devoted to the experience of Orange County, California, in developing a regional trauma system. Chapter Four presents the rationale for development of a trauma registry to describe the epidemiology of trauma and to provide medical accountability of the system. In Chapter Five, Michael Williams discusses the dilemma of authority for designation and presents a detailed description of the designation process, including development of the Request for Proposal (RFP). The financial implications of the system for designated trauma centers as well as for nondesignated hospitals is outlined by Mr. Williams in Chapter Six.

In Chapter Seven, the role of the community hospital is examined by Dr. C. Thomas Thompson, who stresses the importance of a clear understanding and a strong commitment by the board of trustees, the administration, and the medical staff. The complementary role of the university hospital is presented by Dr. Donald D. Trunkey in Chapter Eight, with special emphasis on its role in system direction, teaching, and research.

Having acquired a clear understanding of the issues in trauma system development, the reader will then be prepared to consider the additional clinical and strategic challenges encountered in trauma.

1
PREDICTING THE COMMUNITY'S NEEDS: LOCAL SOLUTIONS TO LOCAL PROBLEMS
Donald D. Trunkey, M.D.

Regionalization of trauma care is currently one of the major efforts of the Committee on Trauma of the American College of Surgeons. The primary reason for this effort is to improve the quality of care for the injured patient. Why then is there so much resistance to this concept? Will a regionalized system truly improve trauma care? If so, how can we predict the community's needs?

Organized regional trauma care had its roots in armed conflict. The Roman legions were probably the first to have designated hospitals for care of war injuries. Larrey's experience with Napoleon's Army provided some of our current models for ambulances and field care. World War I and World War II saw major changes in the delivery of definitive trauma care to the battlefield victim. One of the most dramatic changes, however, occurred during the Korean conflict when the United States Army Medical Corps decided to bypass the battalion aid station and to take the injured soldier directly from the field to the mobile army surgical hospital (MASH). Average time from injury to definitive care during the Korean War was two to four hours, while mortality was kept at a minimum (2.4 percent).

This concept was extended in the Vietnam conflict, where casualties were taken directly from the battlefield to the corps' surgical hospital bypassing the battalion aid station and MASH units. In one study, average time from injury to definitive care was 81 minutes.

Unfortunately, the civilian sector did not apply the principles learned in Korea and Vietnam to care of the injured in the United States. In West Germany, however, they have been applied most efficiently. In 1981 as a James IV Travelling Fellow, I had the opportunity to observe trauma care in six countries.[1]

West Germany has the most impressive system of organized trauma care in the world today. Particularly impressive is their prehospital care, where no patient is more than 30 minutes from a designated trauma center. There is a complete system up and down the Autobahns with rapid transport to the trauma center. Due to a surfeit of physicians within the country, physicians actually go to the accident scene in either ambulances or helicopters. I had a chance to ride in one of the helicopters and was extremely impressed with their response time, efficiency, care at the scene, and timely return to a waiting trauma team. In one case the helicopter was airborne within 2 minutes of the accident and arrived within four minutes, spending only 12 minutes at the scene. The patient, who had extensive long bone fractures, a flail chest, and a closed head injury, was returned to the University of Hanover where he underwent surgery 29 minutes after an accident that occurred 18 kilometers from the hospital. I know of no other country this well organized.

The helicopter system, which is efficiently run by the government, serves as the focus for prehospital care. The average cost per helicopter run is 800 deutche marks ($350). In the past eight years 8,238 flights have been made at the University of Hanover. Eighty-eight percent of these were primary transports; 86 percent of these involved accident cases. The response time averaged 1.4 minutes, and the mean flight distance was 20.8 kilometers. Four thousand seventy-one of the patients were in shock; 532 were agonal. Sixty-two cardiac arrest patients were successfully resuscitated, either at the scene or enroute to the hospital. Of these 62 cardiac arrests, 20 persons left the hospital alive and 19 returned to work. In-transit deaths were less than 0.4 percent. The Germans have also developed a backup system of ground ambulances, which is used when the helicopters cannot fly.

More important than their prehospital system is the integration of trauma care within the hospitals, which have been categorized and designated as to their capability of caring for the trauma patient. There is an inhouse team of trauma surgeons 24 hours a day. These teams include residents, but the attending surgeon is the focus of the team. In Germany, the trauma surgeon is an orthopedic surgeon who has had four years of general surgery and three years of orthopedic surgery, making him eminently qualified to care for over 90 percent of traumatic injuries. The other important members of the trauma team are the neurosurgeon and the anesthesiologist. The trauma surgeon also cares for the patient in the postoperative period, including the intensive care unit. Overall, the care is excellent.

The German system also has a very strong rehabilitation program, the primary goal of which is to get the accident victim back to gainful employment. Although they have not solved the problem of a socialized system in which there are disincentives to return to work, in general their rehabilitation program is second to none.

The area that seems most neglected within the German system is prevention. Drunk driving is a particularly vexing problem and speeds on the German Autobahn are incredible. Penetrating trauma, which is almost nonexistent, reflects a very effective handgun control system in a society that is relatively drug free.

In summary, the German trauma care system is clearly number one in the world today. Since the inception of this integrated system in 1970, the mortality from motor vehicle accidents has experienced a remarkable drop of 25 percent from 16,000 to 12,000 per annum. Assuming that each of these patients returned to gainful employment, made $10,000 a year and paid $2,500 in taxes, this would increase the Gross National Product by $220 million and account for $55 million in taxes. Obviously not everyone returns to work, but the system should more than pay for itself.

During the same period, some regionalized programs have been developed in the United States, most notably in Maryland, Denver, Houston, and more recently in some areas of California, including the Inland Counties, Orange County, and San Francisco County. In general, these programs have confirmed that trauma centers save lives and are cost effective.

There have been several studies that have documented poor outcome when trauma care is not integrated or organized. In 1960, Van Wagoner[2] investigated 606 male soldiers in Texas, concluding that 96 cases would have probably survived had adequate treatment been instituted, and an additional 103 cases would possibly have been salvaged if their treatment had been appropriate. Another study by Frey[3] showed that 28 out of 159 patients who died as a result of injuries were inappropriately treated. In 1972, Gertner[4] showed that one-third of the deaths involving abdominal trauma in the Baltimore area were preventable.

In the San Francisco Bay Area we have performed four studies examining trauma deaths. The first of these compared trauma deaths in San Francisco's trauma center with those in community hospitals,[5] showing that patients from motor vehicle accidents treated in nontrauma hospitals had a significantly higher chance of dying than those treated in the trauma center. The second study, done in conjunction with Dr. John West in Orange County, has been reported in detail elsewhere.[6] A third study done in 1977[7] further documented poor outcome when patients are taken to a nontrauma center. Most recently we have examined trauma care in eight Bay Area counties and have concluded that 40 percent of the patients might have been salvaged if they had not experienced delays in diagnosis or appropriate surgical care.[8]

Numerous other studies have been done in Wisconsin,[9] Vermont,[10] Salt Lake City,[11] and New York,[12] which have shown that the number of preventable deaths attributable to an inadequate system varies from 30 to 40 percent.

A study has recently been completed in Portland, Oregon, by Dr. Dan Lowe at the University of Oregon. Lowe and his colleagues prospectively studied over 700 patients admitted to 23 hospitals in a six-county area, including Portland and the surrounding rural areas. One hundred nineteen of the trauma cases were considered to have had inappropriate care as documented by death or disability. Furthermore, they showed that the average surgeon response time was over one hour.[13] Familiarity with this literature can lead to only one conclusion: trauma centers do make a difference, not only in outcome, but also in the cost to society.

If we accept the premise that trauma centers are desirable, we must then ascertain how many trauma centers are desirable and where they will be located. This will depend on the geography, population density, and local resources.

For every 1 million persons, approximately 1,000 are critically injured in motor vehicle accidents every year and another 9,000 are noncritically injured, based upon statistics from the California Highway Patrol and the Department of Health and Human Services.[14] It has been estimated that it requires 1,000 severely injured patients annually to support a Level I facility, and 350 to 500 severely injured patients to support a Level II facility. The need for Level III facilities will depend on the number of noncritically injured patients in the region.

There are obvious exceptions to these general rules, and the factors that most influence these exceptions are population density and geography. For example, in the Rocky Mountain West it may be impractical to have a Level II or Level I facility outside of the major urban areas of Salt Lake City or Denver. One could rationalize having a Level II in Boise, but, in general, the rural areas will have to rely on earlier recognition and air transport to a Level II or I facility. The rural region more than any other points out that there will never be a perfect system where all severely injured trauma patients will be within a reasonable distance of a Level I or II facility.

Other countries that have encountered similar problems are New Zealand and Australia. In Australia, the flying doctor program in the Outback has proven to be a model for other sparsely populated regions.

In the 1979 document, "Hospital Resources for Optimal Care of the Injured Patient,"[15] the American College of Surgeons recommended that a Level I facility care for a minimum of 1,000 severely injured patients a year, and a Level II facility care for 400. Although these numbers were somewhat arbitrary, they were based on the best data available at the time.

Recently, it has been shown that there is a positive correlation between outcome and the number of cases, indicating that the individual surgeon should manage 50 critical surgical patients a year to maintain his skills and to reduce mortality and morbidity.[16] In a Level I facility, this translates into having eight full-time attendings treating 400 cases a year, with the remaining 600 cases serving as case material for training purposes. In the Level II facility, 400 cases would be adequate for a panel of eight surgeons. Obviously these are guidelines that should not be interpreted as rigid standards but should be considered in light of local needs and resources.

Staffing needs have not been similarly established for emergency physicians or nurses, but maintenance of skills and experience should be equally important for these individuals. Quantitative data in this area must await further studies.

Based on this data, one can assume that there are at least 240,000 critically injured patients in the United States annually. This is actually a conservative estimate, since it does not take into account violent trauma in the large urban areas, nor does it address accidents on the farm, industry, or home. Assuming 240,000 critically injured patients annually, we could easily justify 125 Level I facilities and 300 Level II facilities. Presumably the Level I facilities would be associated with teaching hospitals and would provide the resources for training surgeons, emergency physicians, and nurses. The Level II facilities would be primarily community hospitals geographically distributed throughout the country. This is an ideal scenario and does not recognize the reality of politics. It is also based on relatively soft data and, as in any embryonic program, should serve only as a guideline.

How does one choose which hospital in a community will be the Level I or II facility? There is intense competition for this prestige designation and ideally it should not become part of the strategic arms-like race that has plagued intensive care units and computerized tomography.

The most democratic method of approaching the problem of designation uses the Request for Proposal (RFP) as a tool for measuring commitment and capabilities of competing institutions. Designation of centers can then be made based on objective data that can be evaluated by a review agency or by outside consultants. Centers so designated must then be reviewed periodically to ensure that they continue to fulfill their commitment to the patient and the community.

REFERENCES

1. Trunkey, DD: On the nature of things that go bang in the night. *Surgery* 92(2): 123–32.
2. Van Wagoner, FH: Died in hospital: A three-year study of deaths following trauma. *J. Trauma* 1:184, 1961.
3. Frey, CF, Huelke, DF, Gikas, PW: Resuscitation and survival in motor vehicle accidents. *J. Trauma* 9:292, 1969.
4. Gertner, HR, Baker, SP, Rutherford, RB, Spitz, WU: Evaluation of the management of vehicular fatalities secondary to abdominal injury. *J. Trauma* 12:425, 1972.
5. Trunkey, DD, Lim, RC: Analysis of 425 consecutive trauma fatalities: An autopsy study. *JACEP* 8:368, 1974.
6. West, JG, Trunkey, DD, Lim, RC: Systems of trauma care: A study of two countries. *Arch. Surg.* 114:455, 1979.
7. Baker, CC, Oppenheimer, L, Stephens, B, Lewis, FR, Trunkey, DD: Epidemiology of trauma deaths. *Amer. J. Surg.* 140:144, 1980.
8. Trunkey, DD: Bay Area trauma care. Bulletin, San Francisco Medical Society, p. 22, February, 1982.
9. Detmer, DE, Moylan, JA, Rose, J, Schulz, R, Wallace, R, Daly, R: Regional categorization and quality of care in major trauma. *J. Trauma* 17:592, 1977.
10. Foley, RW, Harris, LS, Pilcher, DB: Abdominal injuries in automobile accidents: Review of care of fatally injured patients. *J. Trauma* 17:611, 1977.
11. Dove, DB, Stahl, WM, Del Guercio, LR: A five-year review of deaths following urban trauma. *J. Trauma* 20:760, 1980.
12. Houtchens, BA: Major trauma in the rural mountain west. *JACEP* 6:343, 1977.
13. Lowe, D: Personal communication, 1982.
14. Simone, B: Personal communication, 1981.
15. Hospital Resources for Optimal Care of the Injured Patient. *Bull. Am. Coll. Surg.* August, pp. 43–48, 1979.
16. Luft, HS, Bunker, JP, Enthouen, AC: Should operations be regionalized? *New Eng. J. Med.* 301:1364, 1979.

2
URBAN SYSTEMS OF TRAUMA CARE: THE BALTIMORE EXPERIENCE
Alasdair Conn, M.D.

Designation of rural trauma facilities differs from urban designation. In the rural area there are typically few hospitals with either Level I or Level II capabilities, so that the primary difficulties are encountered in improving the system of prehospital care. Problems include response times and appropriate use of resources such as helicopters to transport the patient from the scene of the injury to a trauma center as expeditiously as possible. In urban areas the problems tend to be more political.

In typical urban situations, such as Baltimore, there are often a large number of hospitals with potential Level I or Level II capabilities. Within Baltimore, a city of approximately 900,000, there are 14 hospitals, 8 of which can potentially meet the American College of Surgeons (ACS) Level I criteria, while the remaining 6 can potentially meet ACS Level II criteria. In the City of Baltimore the categorization and designation of hospitals followed the process already completed in the rest of Maryland.

Designation was based not only on the availability of resources but also on geography. Helicopters could not be used in the city, so facilities were located to limit transport time to 20 minutes during peak traffic flow. The Maryland Institute for Emergency Medical Services Systems (MIEMSS) receives copies of all ambulance run sheets within the state, from which it was determined that 800 of the city's 80,000 ambulance runs a year could be considered trauma patients. Ideally, this would have required designation of only one or two facilities, but because of constraints in transport, the large number of hospitals potentially able to meet Level I criteria, and political pressures, more than two hospitals were designated. It would have been extremely difficult, for example, not to designate an institution such as Johns Hopkins University as a Level I trauma center. The political consequences of such an exclusion could have been disastrous for the EMS agency.

As a result four hospitals were designated in 1979, including University Hospital, Johns Hopkins Hospital, Sinae Hospital, and Baltimore City Hospitals. Many of these hospitals had already participated in the state EMS system with Johns Hopkins Pediatric Center providing pediatric trauma care, Baltimore City Hospitals Burn Center delivering burn care, and the University of Maryland Hospital functioning as a referral neonatal center. In addition, the Shock Trauma Unit at the University of Maryland continues to function as a resource center for spinal cord injuries.

Considerable political pressure still exists to designate even more trauma centers. One such contending hospital is only six or seven blocks away from Johns Hopkins, but the EMS agency has so far managed to resist these political pressures.

Integral to the success of the trauma system has been the fact that many of the inner city trauma patients have poor financial resources. The romance of becoming a trauma center has thus been balanced by the reality of the bottom line, and some hospitals have chosen to decrease their involvement in the system.

Seminars were conducted for the paramedics of the Baltimore City Fire Department and on November 1, 1979, the program went on-line. Triage criteria included unequal pupils (now being replaced with the Glasgow Coma Scale), blood pressure of less than 80 mm Hg, utilization of the military antishock trousers (MAST) to maintain a blood pressure of 80 mm Hg, gunshot wounds to the chest, and a prolonged period of unconsciousness with external evidence of injury.

Monthly meetings are held with representatives of all of the area-wide trauma centers along with two observers from nondesignated hospitals. Some initial problems with the paramedics were corrected, and the program continues to function reasonably well.

Presently, approximately 70 percent of the trauma identified in the prehospital phase is being transported to the trauma centers. During the first year of study it became clear that prehospital identification of trauma patients is extremely difficult when based on physiological parameters that do not manifest themselves clearly in the five-minute response time typical of urban advanced life support (ALS) units. The majority of injuries have been penetrating wounds with an Injury Severity Score of 15. Accordingly, two modifications have been made in an attempt to increase the accuracy of prehospital triage. The first of these has been to provide direct communication between the paramedic and the trauma medical control physician located at the Shock Trauma Unit. The paramedic on the street can now utilize Med-Channel 6 to consult directly with the trauma surgeon who carries a portable walkie-talkie whenever he or she is on call in the hospital.

The second tool now being implemented is a computerized ambulance run sheet. Information contained in the run sheet previously required manual entry into the computer, but an optically scanned ambulance run sheet is now being developed that will allow entry of 500 cases an hour. The computer will then be able to identify whether a patient falls into the category of trauma and whether he or she was subsequently transported to one of the trauma centers. It is hoped that the trauma communication channel and the computerized ambulance run sheet will help to increase compliance in the prehospital phase.

Long-term planning is now being done by the Department of State Planning, which has agreed to the trauma concept and is responsible for critical review of requests by additional hospitals that wish to improve their emergency rooms or intensive care units for the management of the critically injured.

3
RURAL SYSTEMS OF TRAUMA CARE: THE COLORADO EXPERIENCE
Henry C. Cleveland, M.D.
Dan Dracon, M.D.

The problems of a rural-urban emergency medical services (EMS) system differ from those of a strictly urban system. Rural prehospital care has changed remarkably in the last ten years with the infusion of Department of Transportation (DOT) and Department of Health, Education and Welfare (HEW) monies, which have allowed small towns and facilities to purchase new equipment and train new personnel. Expansion of these resources has resulted in the charge that some rural systems are now overtraining personnel whose skills will eventually deteriorate in the absence of adequate patient volume. I take exactly the opposite view, contending that personnel in rural areas need to be better trained in order to deal effectively with the challenges of long distances and low volume.

One of the problems experienced by small rural communities is their dependence on a single ambulance that may be well equipped and well staffed, but has no backup. Such ambulance services often feel obligated to remain in their own area and may not be interested in driving long distances to deliver injured patients to major urban centers.

From the standpoint of the rural facility, the Colorado experience has been most interesting. In many such towns, the community hospital is served by a small medical staff, which places the individual physicians in an uncomfortable position. While the hospital may not be optimally staffed or equipped to handle trauma patients, it still constitutes the point at which initial triage and stabilization must be instituted. Of primary importance at this stage is the need for the physicians to recognize the existence of a problem that will require additional management at a trauma center. Consequently, they are often anxious to transfer their patients to a more sophisticated center if a transport system can be developed.

The most important part of a rural trauma system is the development of a method of interhospital transfer to simplify the process for referring physicians. If they can be provided with a system that allows them to make a single phone call resulting in the orderly development of all other details (transport, equipment, etc.), they will generally be more than willing to transfer the patient. The initiation of such a transfer rests with the rural physician, who must be able to talk directly with the receiving physician at the trauma center.

When transporting or transferring seriously ill patients, it is essential to consider what personnel and equipment will be required to function as an extension of the trauma center. Choppers are generally used for difficult access or when distances are fewer than 150 miles. In other instances, fixed-wing aircraft are generally most cost effective. In too many cases, however, air transportation systems have been developed without proper attention to the provision of adequate space for the personnel and equipment required for advanced life support (ALS) transport of unstable patients.

Training programs in trauma continue to be popular in rural areas with physicians, emergency medical technicians (EMTs), and dispatchers. Courses in Advanced Trauma Life Support have helped significantly in improving the initial handling of trauma patients before transfer. Equally important have been efforts to train dispatchers to the basic EMT level, providing them with the skills necessary to deal effectively with both physicians and paramedics.

In prehospital trauma care, it is important to develop ALS priorities appropriate for critically injured patients. There is no question about the differences in the management of the injured patient who is located only three to four minutes away from an urban trauma center compared to the patient who suffers an identical injury in a rural region. This concept of "load and go" was initially formulated in an attempt to develop separate prehospital priorities for the urban trauma patient who has historically been treated in the same manner as the critical nontrauma patient. In the urban setting, the team should minimize field time by limiting priorities to the ABCs of basic life support (BLS), splinting and moving the patient as quickly as possible. Rural trauma patients, however, cannot be managed in such a simplistic manner because of longer transport distances that require the provision of ALS for prolonged periods of time.

From the standpoint of evaluation, Dr. Lynn Jacobs has recently completed a study in Boston evaluating the role of the paramedic in the care of the trauma patient. Using a well-constructed and tightly controlled paramedic system, he has evaluated data on paramedic intervention using severity indexes to evaluate outcomes. The study has demonstrated that paramedics make a positive contribution to the treatment of trauma victims, underscoring the importance of continuing support of these field personnel.

Communication must be kept simple. Telemetry should be abolished, although conversations should continue to be taped as they provide an excellent medicolegal and audit record.

Medical control cannot be overemphasized. Although much of the medical control described on paper does not exist in reality, it still constitutes the only extension of the physician in the field. The paramedics must be supported, and the best way to assist them is by assuming medical control of the microphone and communicating with them directly.

Finally, as Dr. Trunkey and others have shown, there is no question that rapid transport systems, such as those developed by the armed services, can also help to save civilian lives.

4
MEDICAL AUDIT OF TRAUMA SYSTEMS
Richard H. Cales, M.D.

Inherent in the development of an emergency medical services (EMS) system is the responsibility of physicians to provide medical accountability of the system and its services. A description of the epidemiology of a condition such as trauma, which constitutes the third leading cause of death in the United States,[1] necessitates implementation of uniform methods of evaluation. In this regard, the medical audit of trauma may be compared to that of cancer, a clinical area in which the development of the registry has had a significant impact on the quality of care.

In this chapter we will examine the objectives, structure, and implementation of the registry as it relates to the medical audit of trauma.

OBJECTIVES OF MEDICAL AUDIT

The medical audit of trauma is a dynamic process that must be designed to meet the evolving requirements of the system (Table 4.1). In regions that are contemplating development of a trauma system, utilization of a trauma registry to audit the quality of care may be used to describe the nature, extent, and significance of problems in trauma care. Specific issues include the number and location of patients, the nature and extent of injury, the availability and appropriateness of care, and outcome. Data obtained from the registry may then be utilized to develop specific recommendations for develop-

Table 4.1   Objectives of Medical Audit of Trauma

Presystem Audit Objectives
Document deficiencies in care
Identify available resources
Develop trauma plan criteria
Postsystem Audit Objectives
Short Range
    Evaluate patient/system care
    Establish system efficacy
Long Range
    Evaluate patient/system care
    Medical research

ment of a trauma system including (1) the number, location, and levels of care (system criteria); (2) medical standards (facility criteria); and (3) patient identification (triage criteria).

Newly established trauma systems are subject to intense political and economic pressures requiring medical audit that provides justification of the system itself in addition to evaluation of the quality of patient care. The trauma registry is especially well suited for such an evaluation, because it provides the comprehensive system data required for medical evaluation of the relationship of system care and outcome. This may be accomplished either by a retrospective comparison of results of pre- and post-system care or, in the event that presystem data is unavailable, by a prospective comparison of patients treated in the system versus those who are not.

It is in the well-established trauma system, however, where questions of justification and efficacy are no longer of overriding concern, that the registry finally settles into its permanent role of medical audit and research.

STRUCTURE OF THE TRAUMA REGISTRY

The trauma registry is a complex tool that, when properly developed, provides a comprehensive data base for describing the interaction of multiple variables in trauma care, including demography, pathology, medical care, and mortality and morbidity. An example of an operational trauma registry appears in Figure 4.1.

A description of the population includes the parameters of age, sex, location, and etiology. Etiologic categorization generally starts with separation of injuries into blunt and penetrating injuries. The majority of blunt injuries are attributed to motor vehicle accidents, including motorcyclists, bicyclists, and pedestrians, although se-

Figure 4.1 Trauma Patient Registry

Trauma patient # _____   Hospital record # _____
Patient name _____   By: _____ R.N.

I. PREHOSPITAL PHASE

A. Identification

    Prehospital log # _____
    Sex: 1 male   2 female
    Age: _____
    Prehospital unit # _____
    Arrive   Leave
    scene _____ hrs scene _____ hrs
    Arrive   Extrication
    hosp. _____ hrs time _____ hrs
    Location _____
                      Street
    _____ _____
         City   Zip

    Type: 01 Auto   07 Gunshot
           02 Motorcycle   08 Stabbing
           03 Bicycle   09 Other penet
           04 Pedestrian   _____
           05 Fall   10 Fire
           06 Other blunt   11 Other
    _____ _____

    Auto: 1. Driver/seatbelt
           2. Driver/no seatbelt
           3. Driver/unknown
           4. Passenger/seatbelt
           5. Passenger/no seatbelt
           6. Passenger/unknown
    Motorcycle: 1. Driver/helmet
                   2. Driver/no helmet
                   3. Driver/unknown
                   4. Passenger/helmet
                   5. Passenger/no helmet
                   6. Passenger/unknown

B. Status

    Vitals: P _____ R _____ BP ___/___
    Blood loss _____ cc
    Injuries: 1. Head/neck
             2. Chest
             3. Abdomen
             4. Extremity
             5. Other _____
    Glasgow Coma Scale:
      Eyes   4 3 2 1
      Motor   6 5 4 3 2 1
      Verbal   5 4 3 2 1
    Total _____
    Pupils: 1. PERRL
           2. Unilateral dilated
           3. Bilateral dilated
           4. Other _____

C. Treatment

Airway:	Cardiac:
1. EOA	1. MAST
2. ET	2. IV
3. Crico	3. CPR
4. Other	4. Other

Vent:	Spine:
1. Assisted	1. Backboard
2. Thoracocentesis	2. C-collar
3. Other	3. Sandbags
	4. Other

D. Disposition

    Field arrest: 1. Yes   2. No
                    Time_____hrs
    Designated by: 1. Paramedics/
                       medical control
                 2. Trauma service/
                   trauma team
               3. Transferred to
                   trauma center

Figure 4.1 Trauma Patient Registry (cont.)

II. EMERGENCY DEPARTMENT PHASE

A. Origin

    Interhospital transfer
        Date arrived _____
        Time arrived _____ hrs
        From _____
        Reason_____
    Field transport
        Date admitted _____
        Time admitted _____ hrs
        Mode: 1. ALS ambulance
                  2. BLS ambulance
                  3. No ambulance
                  4. Helicopter

B. Treatment

    Vitals: Temp _____ Pulse _____
            Resp _____ BP ___/___
    Blood _____ hrs.
    Procedures: 01 Intubation
                  02 Cricothyrotomy
                  03 Tracheostomy
                  04 Assisted ventilation
                  05 Thoracentesis
                  06 Pericardiocentesis
                  07 Peritoneal lavage
                  08 Burr holes
                  09 Thoracotomy
                  10 CPR
    Ancillary: 01 CAT
                  02 Angio

C. Consultations

	Called	Arrived
Tr. Surg.	_____	_____
Anesth.	_____	_____
Neurosur.	_____	_____
Th. Surg.	_____	_____
Orthoped.	_____	_____

D. Admitting Diagnoses

1. _____
2. _____
3. _____
4. _____
5. _____
6. _____

E. Abbreviated Injury Scale (AIS-80)

    External   5 4 3 2 1
    Head   6 5 4 3 2 1
    Neck   6 5 4 3 2 1
    Thorax   6 5 4 3 2 1
    Abdomen 6 5 4 3 2 1
    Spine   6 5 4 3 2 1
    Extremity   4 3 2 1
    ISS: 1. _____
           2. 75 (Automatic with 6)

F. Disposition

1. Expired _____ hrs
2. Sent to OR _____ hrs
3. Admit to ICU _____ hrs
4. Admit to ward _____ hrs
5. Transferred _____ hrs
6. Discharged home _____ hrs

Figure 4.1   Trauma Patient Registry (cont.)

III. OPERATIVE CARE PHASE

A. Admission

   Date admitted to OR _____ Vitals: P_____ BP_____/_____
   Time anesthesia started _____ hrs.   Blood time (if none in ED) _____ hrs.

B. Operations

	Date	ICD-9-CM
_____	_____	_____
_____	_____	_____
_____	_____	_____
_____	_____	_____
_____	_____	_____

IV. ICU PHASE

A. Length of Stay

   Days in ICU _____   Days on respirator _____

B. Complications

01 Shock on admission	06 Cardiac failure	11. Pulmonary infection
02 Myocardial infarct	07 Renal failure	12. Other infections
03 Cardiac arrest	08 Respiratory failure	_____
04 Pulmonary embolus	09 Hepatic failure	13 DIC
05 Stress hemorrhage	10 Wound infection	14 Other _____

V. DISPOSITION

A. Total Length of Stay

   Date of discharge _____   Days in hospital _____

B. Condition on Discharge

   1. Discharged w/preinjury capacity   4. Discharged to convalescent care
   2. Discharged w/temporary handicap   5. Transferred to _____
   3. Discharged w/permanent handicap   6. Death - Autopsy   1 Yes   2 No

C. Discharge Diagnoses:

ICD-9-CM	ICD-9-CM
_____ _____	_____ _____
_____ _____	_____ _____
_____ _____	_____ _____
_____ _____	_____ _____

rious injuries also occur in falls from great heights and in crush injuries such as those seen in industry. Penetrating injuries are usually attributed to gunshot and stab wounds. The registry is also useful for evaluating the effects of seat belts, motorcycle helmets, and other safety equipment.

The pathology of trauma may be coded and quantified. Coding may be accomplished by utilizing the method of the International Classification of Diseases (ICD-9-CM),[2] which provides numerical classification for both diagnosis (tabular codes) and etiology (E-codes). Some systems have gone a step further in the development of their registries by systematically cataloguing injuries according to body system and organ.[3,4]

Injury Severity Scoring (ISS) represents a new evaluation tool that was developed to quantify traumatic injury in order to facilitate comparisons between various treatments and outcomes. Examples include the anatomic approach of the American Association for Automotive Medicine in AIS-80,[5] and the combined anatomic-physiologic scale developed by the American College of Surgeons in its Hospital Trauma Index.[6] A new version that combines both of these methods is reported to be nearing completion.

Quantification of long-term morbidity from trauma includes consideration of disability resulting from the injury and its medical management. Comprehensive evaluation of this rehabilitation potential is of paramount importance in evaluating the efficacy of a trauma system. Factors include length of disability, level of eventual function, and cost. In the event that the patient cannot be returned to the pre-injury level of performance, the length and cost of retraining to a new level of function must be included. The true cost of rehabilitation thus includes not only the direct cost of care, but also the indirect costs of support and lost income. The registry categorizes mortality into those who die at the scene and are not transported to a hospital, those who arrest in the field and are dead on arrival, and those who expire in the hospital.

ELEMENTS IN THE TRAUMA REGISTRY

Medical audit of trauma requires systematic evaluation of each aspect of care starting at the moment of injury and progressing through the prehospital, hospital, and rehabilitation phases. The trauma registry is particularly valuable in this process, because it provides the reviewer with a uniform data base that documents individual elements of care according to objective criteria (Table 4.2).

Table 4.2 Elements in the Trauma Registry

Prehospital Phase
  Protocol Compliance
    Treatment
    Triage
    Transport
  Time Intervals
  Interhospital Transfer

Hospital Phase
  Availability of Resources
    Medical and nursing staff
    Ancillary services
    Blood bank
    Operating rooms
  Appropriateness of Care
    Diagnostic studies
    Therapeutic interventions
    Monitoring
    Rehabilitation
  Injury Severity Scoring

Care in the prehospital phase may be evaluated by measuring adherence to established protocols for treatment, triage, and transport. Issues of concern in the field treatment include prompt application of the ABCs of basic life support in conjunction with judicious fluid resuscitation utilizing intravenous fluids and the pneumatic antishock garment.

The registry may also be utilized to study the appropriateness of triage and transport, since it identifies the elapsed prehospital time and the destination of each trauma victim. Careful review of these time intervals will demonstrate whether or not valuable minutes are being lost in the field, while the appropriateness of triage may be evaluated by examining the occurrence of treatment of minor injuries in trauma centers (false positives) and treatment of major injuries in nontrauma centers (false negatives).

Interhospital transfers of trauma patients, which sometimes represent a system compliance problem, are easily traced through the trauma registry. This group includes patients who require interhospital transfer to a trauma center because of an error in field triage and patients who are appropriately transferred within the trauma system from a Level II or Level III center to a higher level of care.

For patients who have been admitted to the hospital, the registry can be utilized to provide information on facility adherence to system criteria relating to availability and appropriateness of care. Examples include diagnostic procedures (angiography, computerized axial tomography), therapeutic interventions (thoracostomy, peritoneal lavage, etc.), ancillary services (lab, x ray), blood transfusion, and surgical intervention. Indicators of surgical compliance include the availability of surgeons, anesthesiologists, and staffed operating rooms.

In the operative, postoperative, and recuperative phases, the registry continues to provide essential medical data on procedures, monitoring, complications, length of stay, and rehabilitative potential.

The final element in the registry is the Injury Severity Score,[5,6] which provides an objective method of evaluating the appropriateness of outcome.

LEVELS OF AUDIT

The trauma registry provides valuable input in the medical audit of trauma at each level of the system. As depicted in Figure 4.2, these levels are represented by a pyramid, which emphasizes individual

Figure 4.2 Levels of Trauma Audit

PARTICIPANTS		TYPES
EMS SYSTEM (Regional)	REGIONAL EMS SYSTEM	SYSTEM AUDIT
EMS Administrative Staff EMS Medical Director EMS Trauma Consultant EMS Trauma Committee		Medical Control Protocol Compliance
EMS SYSTEM (Subregional)	EMS Subregion A / EMS Subregion B / EMS Subregion C / EMS Subregion D	SYSTEM AUDIT Operations
Designated Trauma Service Non-designated participating hospitals		MEDICAL AUDIT Case Presentation
EMS SYSTEM (Local)	Local Trauma Center A / Local Trauma Center B / Local Trauma Center C / Local Trauma Center D	MEDICAL AUDIT
Medical Staff Trauma Service Committee		Mortality & Morbidity

case management at the local level and system management at the subregional and regional levels.

The forum for medical audit of care at the local level is the trauma committee of the medical staff in the designated trauma center. Here the trauma team can openly, yet confidentially, attempt to improve the quality of care by examining the morbidity and mortality that is occurring on their trauma service.

At the intermediate level is the subregional trauma committee, which provides an opportunity for the nondesignated hospitals to meet with their local trauma center to examine the status of trauma care. At this level it is still appropriate to consider the management of individual cases, but it is done in the context of system audit and medical education, since such multihospital committees are not generally afforded any substantial degree of confidentiality.

The top echelon of medical audit of trauma occurs at the emergency medical services (EMS) regional level where the appropriately constituted medical committees are responsible for overseeing the entire operation with emphasis on system management. This entails review of system statistics, consideration of specific problems raised at the local and subregional levels, and responsibility for determining that all medical and system protocols remain current so that the system can consistently provide state-of-the-art medical care to all trauma victims.

SUMMARY

The trauma registry is a versatile audit tool that may be utilized to define the nature and extent of the problem of trauma, to develop and implement a rational solution to the problem, and to provide medical accountability of the resulting system.

REFERENCES

1. Accidental Death Disability: The Neglected Disease of Modern Society. National Academy of Science/National Research Council, Washington, D.C., 1966.
2. International Classification of Diseases (9th Rev.), Clinical Modification. U.S. Department of Health and Human Services, Washington, D.C., 1980.
3. Boyd, DR, Lowe, RJ, Baker, RJ, Nyhus, LM: Trauma registry: New computer method for multifactorial evaluation of a major health problem. *JAMA* 223:422, 1973.
4. Charters, AC, Bailey, JA: Experience with a simplified trauma registry: Profile of trauma at a university hospital. *J. Trauma* 19:13, 1979.

5. Abbreviated Injury Scale (rev.). American Association for Automotive Medicine. Morton Grove, Illinois, 1980.

6. Hospital Resources for Optimal Care of the Seriously Injured (Trauma Appendices). Bulletin, American College of Surgeons, pp. 31–33, February, 1980.

5
THE TRAUMA CENTER DESIGNATION PROCESS
Michael Williams, M.P.A.

The key to the success of a regional trauma system is development of a defensible designation process. If it can be structured so that medical considerations outweigh political and economic concerns, it will significantly minimize bitterness and improve the chances for acceptance of the final recommendations.

THE DESIGNATING AUTHORITY

One of the recurring dilemmas in the regionalization of trauma relates to the authority for designation. At present there is no single recognized authority for designation. At the federal level, the authority exists only if individual health systems agencies (HSAs) choose to interpret their authority to include regional trauma care. Therefore, in most instances one must look to state, regional, or local governments.

Once the authority for designation has been defined, it should be determined whether or not the authority can be delegated. For example, a board of supervisors may elect to delegate the authority for designation to the local medical or surgical society because of their special medical competence in the area.

In California, the state has delegated the authority for designation to the county boards of supervisors through the Pre-Hospital

---

A special thanks to C. Thomas Thompson, M.D. for his review of the manuscript for this chapter.

Emergency Medical Care Personnel Act of 1982, which authorizes the county or local emergency medical services (EMS) agency to "develop triage and transfer protocols to facilitate prompt delivery of patients to appropriate designated facilities." Additionally, the State EMS Authority, which oversees the provisions of the act, requires the local EMS agency to include standards for trauma facilities as part of its "facility consideration."

More recently the State of Florida, prompted by numerous local jurisdictional squabbles over designation, has adopted legislation that precludes any hospital from calling itself a trauma center unless it is so designated by the State Department of Health Resources.

One note of caution: The issue of authority should not be addressed at the expense of other concerns. It is vitally important that there be a recognized medical basis for the system that can be understood by both the medical community and the public, for without such a foundation any designation process will become mired in political and legal challenges.

THE SELECTION PROCESS

Once a community has conceptualized a regional trauma system, developed a plan of action, and approved specific criteria for trauma centers, it is ready for the actual process of designation. In urban/suburban areas it is possible that several hospitals will have the potential to meet or exceed the criteria, while in rural areas there may be none. In the latter situation, the designating body may be required to approach adjoining areas in order to obtain the necessary resources to develop a system. In either case a selection process must be initiated in which the proposed competition will be commensurate with the number and the potential capabilities of the applicants.

During the planning process the designating body should insist on a fair, objective, and medically based selection process. This is generally recognized as consisting of four components: (1) acceptance of applications; (2) presentation of recommendations; (3) defense of recommendations; and (4) provisional and final designations.

It is difficult to predict the exact format of a selection process that will be appropriate for each individual community, because of the multiplicity of needs and resources. Most objective reviews, however, will include the following elements:

- Development of the Request for Proposal (RFP)
- Screening of proposals by staff to ensure minimum standards

- Review of proposals by an objective selection committee of clinical experts
- On-site visits by the selection committee
- Public hearings and appeals
- Provisional designation of hospitals
- Resurvey in six to twelve months
- Final designations

The actual criteria and selection process should be agreed to by all potential applicants and by the designating body prior to the solicitation of applications.

THE SELECTION COMMITTEE

Ideally, an impartial selection committee would be composed entirely of clinical experts in trauma chosen from outside the region. Following appointment, it would be vested with total authority to make recommendations for designation based solely on the medical capabilities and commitments of the applicants.

The more noncritical or marginal experts that are added to the selection committee, the greater will be the chance for political influence on the process. This is particularly true if the actual designating body is a nonmedical entity such as a board of supervisors.

THE REQUEST FOR PROPOSAL

A Request for Proposal (RFP), which is commonly utilized in the solicitation of trauma proposals, is a process for choosing the hospital that best meets the system's requirements and promotes the best care. The RFP process has the additional advantage of stimulating competition, which in some areas has led to applications that significantly exceed minimum criteria.

The RFP process should be perceived as occurring in two stages: the written proposal and the on-site survey. A written proposal should be solicited that accurately describes the hospital's capabilities and commitment. The selection committee should allot adequate time to scrutinize and to discuss the written application prior to the on-site survey. The committee will then be adequately prepared to verify the written proposal during the actual on-site survey.

The following components should be reflected in written RFP:

- A basic description of the region's trauma problem (this indirectly describes the applicant hospital's understanding of the region's needs)

- A conceptual overview of how the applicant hospital will address the system and its problems
- A description of how the applicant hospital meets the criteria, indicating in the case of exceptions how the exceptions will affect the quality of care
- A specific description of new commitments being made by the applicant and how they will differ from the normal operation of the hospital
- A statement as to why the applicant should be selected over other hospitals
- Specific information based on the hospital's perception of the selection process

THE ON-SITE SURVEY

Sixty percent of the applicant hospital's score will probably be determined during the on-site survey, largely due to the lasting impressions, both positive and negative, that occur when the selection committee meets with the people who will eventually operate the trauma center. If there is a need for a hospital to develop its written proposal properly, then it is doubly important for it to prepare adequately for the on-site survey. Failure to do so may result in the situation in which an applicant hospital submits a superior written application only to lose the designation during the on-site survey because of a lack of staff familiarity with the proposal or because of open staff disagreement as to the extent of hospital commitment.

The on-site survey provides the reviewers with the opportunity to verify the commitments made in the proposal through direct conversations with responsible individuals, including the board of directors, administration, and medical staff. Since a thorough review of equipment and medications is an integral part of the survey, the team should include at least one representative who is familiar with the technical requirements of the criteria (surgical trays, intravenous equipment, autotransfusers, pneumatic antishock trousers, etc.). Particular care should be exercised to ensure that the equipment is readily accessible, and that the staff on duty knows how to utilize it properly.

On-site surveyors should interview all affected departments within the hospital to assess the specific commitments and changes that are occurring (training, data collection, new equipment, etc.). They should also interview on-duty clinical staff, since these individuals are less likely to have rehearsed answers as to the hospital's commitment and understanding of the system. For this reason the survey team may wish to schedule a portion of the on-site survey late in the evening or on the weekend, when trauma patients are more likely to arrive at the hospital. Table 5.1 lists some questions that may be asked of hospital staff.

THE SCORING SYSTEM

Survey teams often utilize a scoring system for evaluating applications, thereby providing the capability of quantifying otherwise

Table 5.1 Trauma Center Designation Site Visit Typical Questions

Board of Directors/Trustees
Describe your commitment to the trauma center concept. If the center began to lose significant dollars, would your board be prepared to add resources?

Administrator
Describe the organizational hierarchy of the trauma program in the hospital. Why do you want this designation? Are you prepared to provide the necessary clinical and administrative staff necessary to support this program? Will you cooperate with regional data collection, training programs, etc.?

Trauma Nurse Coordinator
Describe the training programs you have instituted that directly relate to trauma. To whom do you report?

Chief of Staff
Describe the level of medical staff awareness and commitment to this program. What opposition did you have to this idea?

Trauma Chief
Describe the clinical treatment of a trauma patient in your hospital. How do you monitor clinical care? What are your duties? How much time will you commit to this program? How high a priority is the trauma service in the hospital?

Emergency Department Director
What steps did you take to prepare for this designation? How do you feel about the new role of the trauma surgeon in the ED? (Have you dealt with this?)

On-Duty Intensive Care Unit Nurse
What training programs have you taken recently which are related to trauma? It's 1:00 A.M. and two new trauma patients need to be admitted to the ICU. The ICU is full. Whom do you call?

Lab Technologist
You are asked for 2 units of O negative blood (not typed or crossed). How would you respond?

On-Duty Emergency Department Nurse
What changes have you seen relative to this application? Do you know the indications for the use of an autotransfuser? Please set up a MAST suit. Describe what is on an open thoracotomy tray.

On-Duty Operating Room Nurse
Do you have trouble obtaining stat lab results? How effectively does radiology respond to your needs?

Source: EMS System Design, Irvine, CA.

subjective data. This system can be of special benefit in cases where individual applications exceed (or fail to meet) minimum criteria. Care should be exercised to ensure that such a scoring system does not become an end in itself, but rather that it is utilized as a means to simplify the development of a final conclusion.

The components of such a scoring system are outlined in Table 5.2. One should note the low priority of equipment versus the high priority given commitment, system conceptualization, and patient care. Percentages may be assigned to each main category and subcategory, as in the following example (extracted from Table 5.2):

1. Physician Staffing (30 percent of total score)
    A. Trauma surgeons (25 percent of physician staffing score)
    B. Anesthesiologists (25 percent of physician staffing score)
    C. Specialists (25 percent of physician staffing score)
    D. Emergency physicians (25 percent of physician staffing score)

THE IMPACT OF COMPETITION

The level of competition in a trauma center designation process will depend on the number of qualified applicants. If there were a selection process that kept hospitals from aggressively competing against each other, it would avoid much of the long-term bitterness that is evoked by a highly competitive process.

From the standpoint of quality, however, competition may be helpful because it encourages applicant hospitals to strengthen their commitments. Therefore, the key to a successful designation process is to develop a blend of competition and commitment that precludes long-term hostility and ensures that hospitals make commitments that they are reasonably able to keep.

In the bidding process, it should be understood that it is not necessarily sufficient for an applicant hospital to state that it will meet minimum criteria; it should attempt to exceed criteria in any area that would make a positive contribution to patient care. Nor is it sufficient for an applicant to state that it will begin its commitment on the day of designation; the truly competitive hospital will implement its trauma proposal as early as possible in order to provide the necessary experience and track record to demonstrate its stated commitment.

It should also be understood that competition does not end with designation. Chosen facilities should be required to defend their se-

Table 5.2 Trauma Center Selection Criteria Scoring System/Evaluation Tool

Each of the following components is evaluated on a scale of 0 to 4:
- (0) unacceptable
- (1) below criteria
- (2) meets criteria
- (3) exceeds criteria
- (4) substantially exceeds criteria

I. **PHYSICIAN STAFFING**
   A. Trauma Surgeons
      1. Past experience and training
      2. ACLS/ATLS training
      3. Specific trauma experience
      4. Availability (inhouse)
   B. Anesthesiologists
      1. Past experience and training
      2. ACLS/ATLS training
      3. Availability (inhouse)
   C. Subspecialists
      1. Representation
      2. Availability
   D. Emergency Physicians
      1. Past experience and training
      2. ACLS/ATLS

II. **ADMINISTRATIVE STRUCTURE**
   A. Director
      1. Training/background and trauma experience
      2. Administrative experience
      3. Time commitment
   B. Nurse Coordinator
      1. Training/background and trauma experience
      2. Administrative experience
      3. Time commitment
   C. Structure
      1. Medical control
         a. conceptualization
         b. role designation of trauma team
         c. authority over resources
      2. Administrative control
         a. conceptualization
         b. job descriptions
         c. access to authority structure
      3. Trauma committee
         a. relationship to medical staff/administration
         b. description of authority, roles, etc.
      4. Regional trauma committee
         a. composition
         b. function

Table 5.2 Trauma Center Selection Criteria Scoring System/Evaluation Tool (cont.)

- D. Cost Effectiveness
  1. Administrative overhead
  2. Cost/bed
  3. Capital expenditures
  4. Operative costs
  5. Conceptualization of operational costs/revenue source

III. **TRAUMA SYSTEM CONCEPTUALIZATION**
  - A. Area Description
    1. Proposed catchment area (area, population)
    2. Ability to service area (mode)
    3. Potential volume (growth)
  - B. Patient Management
    1. Medical supervision/orders
    2. Protocols/decision pathways
    3. Priority for trauma patient
  - C. Training
    1. Team development
    2. Physician/nurse training
    3. Regional trauma education
  - D. Evaluation
    1. Criteria
    2. Additional conceptualization; refinement of criteria
  - E. Other
    1. Transfer agreements
    2. Responsibility to indigent patient
    3. Monitoring/recordkeeping

IV. **FACILITY**
  - A. Emergency Department
    1. Overall capacity/beds
    2. Trauma room (dedicated)
    3. Emergency room volume
    4. Equipment
       a. criteria
       b. other (transfuser)
  - B. Operating rooms
    1. Availability
       a. total number
       b. availability (dedicated)
    2. Equipment
       a. criteria
       b. cardiac pump team
       c. full body scanner
       d. other (transfuser, microscope)
  - C. Intensive Care Units
    1. MD staffing
    2. RN staffing
       a. ratio
       b. registry

Table 5.2 Trauma Center Selection Criteria Scoring System/Evaluation Tool (cont.)

       3. Occupancy rate
       4. Equipment
          a. criteria
          b. other
       5. Hyperalimentation protocol
    D. Supportive Services
       1. Radiology
          a. services
             i) criteria
             ii) CAT scan
          b. priority system
          c. MD staffing
       2. Pathology
          a. services
             i) criteria
             ii) other
          b. priority system
          c. blood bank
          d. MD staffing
          e. technologist staffing
       3. Cardiology
          a. technologist staffing
       4. Respiratory
          a. technician staffing

V. SPECIALIZED PROGRAMS
    A. Rehabilitation Program
    B. Psych/Social Service
       1. Staff
       2. Patient
       3. Family
       4. Recovery program
    C. Data Collection System
    D. Monitoring/Evaluation
       1. Grand rounds
       2. Mortality and Morbidity conferences
       3. Other
    E. Public Education/Prevention Program
    F. Other

VI. REGIONAL EMS NEEDS
    A. Relationship with Prehospital System
    B. History of Applicant regarding EMS System Needs
    C. Willingness to Participate in Regional Program
       (data collection, evaluation, training, etc.)
    D. Overall Applicant Potential to Enhance Total EMS System's Needs

VII. OTHER
    A. Individual System Requirements Should Be Added Here.

Source: EMS Systems Design, Irvine, CA

lection on a regular basis even after the formal title has been bestowed.

THE COMMUNITY POLITICAL SETTING

If a designation process were totally fair, objective, and medically based, community politics would not play a part in the designation process for trauma centers. The reality in most communities, however, is that politics does play a part in the process. Unfortunately, its direction and impact are not usually known until it is too late to counteract the effects.

The level of community political activity on this issue will be directly related to the competency of the decision-making body and the stature and credentials of the selection committee. Every effort should be made to ensure a fair, impartial, and unbiased process that is designed to avoid complicated political and legal challenges.

Trauma center development will not occur in every community, and in those areas where it does materialize it may not be appropriate to encourage all hospitals to develop an application to participate in the system. However, the conceptual framework of developing a regional trauma center system may be applied to many other programs and clinical categories, and the proposed implementation model can be applied to other EMS system activities.

SUMMARY

The trauma center issue forces individual jurisdictions to take an inventory of health care priorities, medical commitments, and future directions for the potential benefit of the injured patient. Such an approach is critical in the improvement of trauma care.

6
FINANCIAL CONSIDERATIONS
Michael Williams, M.P.A.

As the fervor to develop trauma centers increases, many hospital administrators and medical staffs are being forced to decide whether or not to participate in the system. To make such a decision adequately requires a thorough understanding of relevant issues inside and outside the hospital. Internal factors include medical staff commitment, existing capabilities in emergency and trauma care, bed capacity, staffing, and most importantly, the financial impact. External factors include assessment of the competition and the method of selection.

This chapter will attempt to provide a fundamental understanding of the financial impact of the system on the individual hospital, whether or not it chooses to participate.

ASSESSMENT OF FINANCIAL ISSUES

The technology for assessing the broad range of influences affecting the financial considerations of trauma center designation has not yet been developed with great precision. Part of this difficulty is attributable to a lack of adequate experience with existing centers. Second, no two hospitals are alike in their priorities or styles of operation. Therefore, each hospital should develop its own rationale for making such a decision.

Certain issues tend to appear repeatedly in discussion with hospitals making a decision to become a trauma center.

- The length of stay for trauma patients is considerably longer than average (15 days).
- The length of stay in the intensive care unit (ICU) is longer than average (4 to 6 days).
- Utilization is high for lucrative ancillary services (lab, x ray, respiratory, pharmacy).
- Utilization is improved for services that are otherwise underutilized on evening and night shifts (60 percent of trauma occurs from 9 P.M. to 3 A.M.).
- Some hospitals have found the patient mix to be better than that of the average emergency patient.
- In areas with trauma systems, the designated centers have benefitted from over triage of trauma patients (12 percent in Orange County; 25 percent in Baltimore).
- Depending on patient mix, applicants have often projected an increase in their profit margin of between 4 to 18 percent.

Indirect financial considerations include the potential for growth of the hospital and its services.

- Many hospitals believe the trauma designation to be but one of a limited number of regional designations, with each designation enhancing the opportunity for obtaining another, e.g., burn center.
- Increased utilization of beds and ancillary services results in the ability to justify expanded services later.
- A trauma center is better able to fit the profile of the successful certificate of need applicant because of its participation in a program that is regionally designated and that reduces duplication by optimizing utilization.

One of the most important assets of a designation, however, is believed to relate to image.

- Trauma centers have the potential to increase other services as a result of their trauma image (one Orange County emergency department has experienced a 12 percent increase in volume along with a significant increase in elective surgeries).
- The designation provides an excellent opportunity for image enhancement, which will assist in nurse and physician recruitment, obtaining research grants, fund raising, and human interest stories.
- The trauma team concept will exhibit a carryover effect on other functions within the hospital, thus enhancing interdisciplinary capabilities.

ASSESSMENT OF FINANCIAL IMPACT

Objectivity is the key to successful assessment of the financial impact of trauma center designation on a hospital. Most hospitals have a tendency to overestimate their overall capability, thereby underestimating the necessary changes that may result in inaccurate cost projections.

The hospital's philosophy, priorities, and long-range goals must be critically analyzed for compatibility with the trauma center concept. Hospitals that provide general acute care while avoiding tertiary care services should take a second look before proceeding with the trauma issue. Hospitals that have a well-respected care capability but that have not previously engaged in a competitive application may also wish to opt out of the process.

In general, a typical community hospital that already excels in its 24-hour emergency and surgical capability will have a solid foundation on which to prepare to meet either local or national trauma standards. Few staffing changes will be required, except in the area of surgical coverage and in volume-related clinical staff. The trauma commitment will additionally require a reorganization and reprioritization of the hospital's staffing and resources.

For those with less than this capability, the trauma commitment may have a significant impact on the hospital, especially in staffing of the operating room and ancillary services.

Physical Plant

Several areas are of paramount importance in assessing total financial impact.

- Trauma resuscitation area
- Operating room(s)
- Intensive care unit(s)
- Medical/surgical beds
- Rehabilitation

This component of the assessment should take into account the existing trauma load of the hospital compared with that of the anticipated volume. Particular emphasis should be placed on the time of day the patient arrives. National experience suggests that 50 to 60 percent of serious trauma occurs between 9 P.M. and 3 A.M. For a busy operating room in which most elective cases end by 6 P.M., the demands on the physical plant will thus be more readily absorbed. A skilled operating room supervisor is a valuable asset in assuring that a suite is immediately available for a trauma admission, even during a busy elective schedule.

Other plant considerations include space for the additional management created by the trauma service and for the additional training staff required by the new clinical service.

Staffing

Financial concerns with respect to staffing may be broken down into three general categories, including management, clinical, and recruitment and training.

Exact management needs will vary, as will specific reimbursement patterns. An example of a community hospital team in Southern California seeing 300 to 400 trauma patients a year includes a trauma physician director (quarter-time, $40,000/year) and a trauma nurse coordinator (fulltime, $35,000/year, including benefits). Job descriptions for these positions are shown in Table 6.1.

From the clinical staffing standpoint, most additional requirements will be volume related, so the costs will be offset by patient revenue. For example, ICU staffing is dependent on the number and severity of patients. In the respiratory therapy department, the number of therapists on each shift is gauged by the number of treatments and the number of patients on ventilators.

A more difficult problem is that of minimum staffing requirements. If the hospital has normally staffed the laboratory with one medical technologist on the night shift, it will not suffice if even one trauma patient is seen, given the demands of stat tests and blood banking.

The third area of concern is recruitment and training costs. In some areas of the country that are experiencing personnel shortages, these costs may be significant and must be recognized in any assessment of financial impact.

Potential Competition

Depending on the proposed designation process, interhospital competition can substantially impact the cost of eventual designation. While local criteria may require a minimum level of hospital commitment as a condition of designation (15-minute, on-call availability of the surgeon), a competitive bidding process between two hospitals may force one hospital to exceed the criteria (24-hour, in-house surgical coverage) to increase its chances of being designated.

Table 6.1 Trauma Program Job Descriptions

Trauma Director
Qualifications
  Experienced, board-certified, general/thoracic surgeon with demonstrated clinical, administrative, and leadership competencies
Responsibilities
  Plan, develop, implement, and direct the trauma center program to meet the needs of critically injured patients.
Duties
  Coordinate the trauma service plan and review the performance of care for trauma patients.
  Assist the trauma committee in establishing quality assurance programs and audits of trauma cases.
  Assist the trauma committee with the development of policies and procedures for a multidisciplinary team approach to care of the trauma patient.
  Establish rapport and coordinate efforts with emergency department, surgery, intensive care unit, laboratory, pharmacy, radiology, respiratory therapy, and other appropriate areas of services.
  Recruit and assume responsibility for qualified trauma surgical physician coverage.
  Chair the trauma committee and regional trauma advisory committee and maintain liaison with area hospitals.
  Supervise the development of training for all trauma team members.
  Assist in the development/monitoring of appropriate prehospital triage criteria.
  Develop/implement trauma operational protocols.
  Maintain liaison with other regional trauma centers.
  Assume responsibility for accuracy and validity of the trauma statistics.
  Develop written transfer agreements as appropriate to include secondary critical-care transport mechanisms.
  Conduct and coordinate research on trauma.
  Organize and conduct grand rounds, morbidity and mortality conferences, and medical audits on trauma patients.
  Act as liaison with regional disaster planning efforts.

Trauma Nurse Coordinator
Qualifications
  Licensed registered nurse with certified emergency nurse (CEN) or certified critical care registered nurse (CCRN) certification with demonstrated abilities as follows:
    Strong critical care/emergency department background
    Leadership qualities
    Good communication skills
    Guided assertiveness
    Goal orientation
    Educational program coordination
Responsibilities
  Responsible for overall staff education, patient-care problem identification, and staff activity coordination with the trauma director.
Duties
  Assess areas of education and performance skills requiring development and establish the priorities with individual trauma team members.
  Staff and coordinate the trauma committee and regional trauma advisory committee meetings.

Table 6.1 Trauma Program Job Descriptions (cont.)

Maintain the trauma registry, including gathering statistics and data.
Assist staff members in the maintenance of advanced trauma life support specialty certifications.
Identify patient education needs for incorporation in community service projects and regional educational programs.
Participate in establishing and coordinating the trauma treatment and operation protocols and policies.
Maintain communication with prehospital personnel and hospital; coordinate trauma matters.
Coordinate liaison of support services.
Coordinate public education/prevention programs.

Source: EMS Systems Design, Irvine, CA.

The list of possibilities is endless by which a hospital could exceed the criteria either to enhance its chances for designation or merely to improve on the program requirements. Other areas include:

- Specialized trauma training programs for physician, nursing, and ancillary service personnel
- Staff field visits to other centers
- Trauma fairs or skill centers
- Public education/prevention programs
- A dedicated trauma ICU
- Sophisticated data collection systems
- Helicopter and helipad capability
- Comprehensive rehabilitation services
- Special trauma eligibility and discharge planners
- Specialized trauma psych/social services
- Trauma postinjury recovery programs
- Pre- or interhospital trauma ambulances
- Special public relations and marketing campaigns

Patient Mix and Demographics

Of major importance in any review of financial impact is the patient insurance mix. Given the expenses identified in the previous sections, this area of assessment will largely determine how much of a financial benefit or burden a hospital will experience with a trauma program. Hospitals with a significant welfare and "no pay" patient mix will require heavy subsidies for the trauma program, while significant proportions of commercial insurance coverage will provide welcome revenue resources for the hospital.

The key to this issue is an accurate evaluation of the existing trauma patient mix as compared with the anticipated mix from any

Financial Considerations

new areas. Of particular importance here is the potential of the trauma program to expand the hospital's catchment or service area into a more lucrative or economically stable area.

CONDUCTION OF A PATIENT PROFILE AND PROJECTION

To assess current hospital financial experience with trauma adequately it is desirable to complete a 12-month trauma profile. If the data base can be widened to include multiple hospitals, more confidence may be placed in the results. Before the methodology for such a profile is developed, however, an exhaustive search should be made for available sources of data.

- Existing hospital/emergency department studies
- Special emergency medical services (EMS) regional studies.
- Hospital council/medical society sources
- Health Systems Agency (HSA) resources
- Peer Standards Review Organization (PSRO) resources
- State and local police data

One methodology used for producing a hospital profile is as follows:

1. Select a physician evaluation team of surgeons and emergency physicians.
2. Identify a patient triage or severity standard, such as the American College of Surgeons standard,[1] the Champion Triage Index,[2] or a local standard.
3. Request all hospital records for the most recent 12-month period available, representing patients with primary ICD-9-CM discharge diagnoses between 800 and 959. (Subsets or specific diagnoses may be selected to decrease the resulting volume of charts.)
4. Have the physician team review each record to determine whether or not the patient meets the criteria selected in step 2. (Care should be taken to identify patients who present as trauma patients in the prehospital phase even though their condition may improve prior to admission. This will ensure an accurate profile of patients who may be sent directly to a trauma center, bypassing the nearest hospital.) Certain prevalent injuries may require special review. For example, concussions (ICD 850) may require an arbitrary standard of a three-day hospital stay to qualify as a major trauma patient. Likewise, many hip

fractures in the elderly are from minor falls and do not constitute multiple system trauma.
5. Once the patients who meet criteria have been identified, the hospital's financial staff should be asked to summarize the information in Table 6.2 for each patient.

This information will be of major assistance in the financial assessment of the potential impact of increasing the hospital's commitment to the trauma patient. The findings of a typical Northern California community hospital of 200 beds serving a middle-to-upper-income population are summarized in Table 6.3.

These data represent trauma from the hospital's existing service area. While no concise methodology exists for predicting the insurance mix of new trauma, certain indexes are available. One such index is the comparison of demographic data for the existing service area to data for the proposed service area. Sources for data (average income, housing value, expendable income indexes, rate of unemployment) vary greatly by area, but include:

- 1980 census
- Chamber of Commerce
- County/city planning departments
- Newspaper/radio/TV marketing studies
- Health system agencies
- Regional government agencies/associations
- Hospital market research
- Hospital council

Care should be exercised to compare data gathered from the same year to ensure consistency. Table 6.4 represents an example of such an assessment by a Northern California hospital, suggesting that the economic status of the potential new patient would deteriorate slightly by extending the service area. The existing service area, however, appears to be very economically stable.

An example of patient insurance mixes with available comparable demographic data is listed in Table 6.5.

PROFILE OF A TYPICAL COMMUNITY HOSPITAL

It should be understood that development of a data base on the financial implications of trauma is very much an individual hospital issue. Broad multihospital comparisons may not take into account the strengths and weaknesses of individual hospitals, resulting in an unpredictable effect on cost. Some of these variables include:

Table 6.2 Trauma Center Patient Financial Profile

Etiology
  Mechanism (blunt or penetrating)
  Specific diagnosis
Demographics
  Employed (yes/no)
  City of residence
  Age and sex
  Day and time of arrival
  Manner of arrival
Insurance Coverage (by category)
Length of Stay
  Total
  ICU
  Med/surg
  Rehabilitation
Average Bills by Cost Center
Billings
  Total
  Government allowances
  Other write-offs (estimate for open accounts)

Table 6.3 Composite of Trauma Financial Profile for a Community Hospital in Northern California

	No.	%
Total Number of Patients	122	
Payment Mechanism		
Commercial	77	63.1
Medicare	14	11.5
Patient Pay	9	7.4
MediCal	8	6.6
Workman's Comp	8	6.6
HMO	3	2.5
Cash	2	1.6
Champus	1	0.8
Time of Arrival		
0–3:00 hrs.	7	5.7
3:01–6:00 hrs.	4	3.3
6:01–9:00 hrs.	11	9.0
9:01–12:00 hrs.	11	9.0
12:01–15:00 hrs.	14	11.5
15:01–18:00 hrs.	23	18.9
18:01–21:00 hrs.	25	20.5
21:01–24:00 hrs.	10	8.2
Unknown	17	13.9

Table 6.3 Composite of Financial Profiles Community Hospital of Northern California (cont.)

	No.	%
Injury		
Penetrating	11	9.0
Blunt	111	91.1
Mechanism of Injury		
Motor Vehicle	72	59.0
Violent crime	12	9.8
Fall	20	16.4
Other/unknown	18	14.8
Month of Arrival		
Jan.	16	13.1
Feb.	10	8.2
March	16	13.1
April	12	9.8
May	12	9.8
June	9	7.4
July	12	9.8
Aug.	11	9.0
Sept.	3	2.5
Oct.	7	5.7
Nov.	8	6.6
Dec.	8	6.6
Employment		
Yes	63	51.6
No	59	58.4
Age Composition Years		
0–09	8	6.6
10–14	2	1.6
15–19	16	13.1
20–30	36	29.5
31–40	17	13.9
41–50	14	11.5
51–60	12	9.8
61 +	17	13.9
City of Residence		
City A		40.3
City B		8.1
City C		8.1
City D		6.5
City E		4.0

Financial Considerations

Table 6.3 Composite of Financial Profiles Community Hospital of Northern California (cont.)

	No.	%
City F		3.2
City G		2.4
City H		1.6
Other county		13.3
Other out of county		8.9
Out of state		1.6

Total Billings
ICU/SCU	$118,000
Med/Surg/Peds/Gen.	169,500
Acute rehabilitation	66,500
Ancillaries	364,500
	$718,500

Average Patient Bill
$5,889

Average Lengths of Stay
Med/Surg	8.8	days
Acute rehab	2.9	days (for acute rehab. patients, 61.2 days)
ICU	1.9	days (for ICU patients, 3.5 days)
Total	12.7	days

Note: Total charts reviewed; 452. Total cases meeting criteria; 122. Dates of sample; 5/80–6/81.

- Availability of trained, committed trauma surgeons
- Current adequacy of the emergency department
- Unique physical plant considerations
- Nurse and paraprofessional shortages
- Level of interhospital competition
- Degree of medical staff interest
- Volume and frequency of current trauma and major surgical cases
- Other hospital priorities and goals that may enhance or detract from the trauma program

While specific comparisons should be made cautiously with regard to the experience of other hospitals, a hospital profile may be made to provide direction to hospitals reviewing this issue. For this purpose two formats may be utilized. Table 6.6 lists patient attributes that may have an impact on the financial viability of a trauma program. Table 6.7 is a summary of a start-up and opera-

Table 6.4 Economic Indicators of Existing and Projected Trauma Service Area for a Northern California Hospital

Service Area	Population	Median Annual Income	Median Housing Unit Value	Median Contract Rent	Percent Housing Unit Overcrowded
Current:					
Partial Area A and Area B:	81,148	$41,265	150,300	346	.03
Proposed Area:					
Remainder of Area A	22,852	54,265	158,365	329	.02
Remainder of Area B	39,978	38,180	130,876	338	.03
North	81,883	21,100	96,209	299	.10
North Central	108,362	31,320	113,000	308	.05
South Central	104,166	40,050	133,300	300	.04
South	71,895	39,128	127,800	302	.08
Coast	48,552	23,450	104,100	340	.04
Other	28,493				
Total	587,329				

Source: 1980 Census.

Table 6.5 Trauma Payment Mechanism Survey: Nine California Hospitals

	Hospital Type	Number of Beds	Patients	Population*	Median Effective Buying Income†	County Median Effective Buying Income	Median Home Sales Value‡
A	Community	400	83	793,018	17,227	18,680	66,277
B	Community	135	35	88,292	20,868	—	68,537
C	Community		102	223,506	18,505	—	84,861
D	University	878	207	404,390	16,210	—	81,569
E	Community	256	87	155,059	16,777	—	54,113
F	Community	312	91	275,553	19,266	—	85,484
G	Community	128	45	210,557	16,264	16,763	139,678
H	Community	250	122	81,148	21,105	—	150,300
I	Community	500	204	92,904	17,118		

Total Patients Reviewed: 976

*1979 Data, Sales and Marketing Management, 1980
†1980 Census data
‡1978 Data, real estate boards
Source: EMS Systems Design, Irvine, CA

Table 6.5 Trauma Payment Mechanism (cont.)

Payment Mechanism (%)

Commercial	Medical	Medicare	Cash	Comp	Other
51	26	11	2	10	—
71	6	14	3	6	—
53	25	5	7	—	9
71	14	13	1	—	—
40	24	13	13	—	11
46	12	26	2	8	5
67	13	7	2	1	7
63	7	14	2	7	4
47	19	9	19	—	7

Table 6.6 Trauma Patient Parameters: 1980–1981 Survey of 958 California Trauma Patients

Sex
  Male   75%
  Female 25%

Age
  65% of the patients were between the ages of 15–24

Employment
  Yes 37%
  No 63% (reflects school-age victims with parental insurance)

Time of arrival
  60% arrived after 9:00 P.M. and before 3:00 A.M.

Day of arrival
  Thursday   19%
  Friday   22%
  Saturday   24%
  All other days 35%

Month of arrival
  Varies—vacation areas experienced an increase during summer months

Average length of stay
  Med/Surg. 11   days
  ICU   4.5 days
  Rehab.   8   days

Average patient bill
  $11,500

Percent of bill attributed to ancillaries
  55%

Patient insurance mix
  Varies—tended to be as good or a better mix than existing emergency room patients

Source: EMS Systems Design, Irvine, CA

tional budget for a typical community hospital. In evaluating the data, several comments are in order.

- Costs are not represented that are currently integrated into the patient revenue system, e.g., new ICU nurses.
- If local standards require an inhouse surgeon or anesthesiologist, a guarantee against billings may be required. Some hospitals have guaranteed each specialist as much as $1,000 per day for this coverage. However, if patient volumes are adequate, most hospitals will not be required to pay this guarantee.
- No costs are included for program enhancement (public education, data collection, research projects) that may be required due to competition in the application process or because of a hospital's commitment to the program. Often there are existing hospital resources for these programs.
- No costs are included for those hospitals that implemented staffing changes to enhance an application or to develop a "track re-

Table 6.7 Startup/Operating Budget—Typical Community Trauma Center

Start-up Budget	
Remodel Resuscitation Area	$150,000
Overhead X ray—ED	60,000
Application Development	10,000
Equipment Costs	
Major	
Monitor defibrillator ED	6,500
Pressure monitor ED	9,000
Auto B/P monitor ED	1,700
Radiographic stretcher	3,600
Minor	
Assorted surgical instruments	2,000
Pediatric equipment	1,500
Training	
(Special program for nurses/physicians)	10,000
Office space for Trauma Director/Coordinator	5,000
Total Start-up Costs	$259,300
Annual Operating Budget	
Trauma Director Quarter-time	$ 40,000
Nurse Coordinator	38,000
Clerk	18,000
Supplies & Printing	15,000
Marketing	5,000
Total Annual Costs	$116,000

Source: EMS Systems Design, Irvine, CA

cord," e.g., 24-hour operating room coverage prior to designation and its increased volume.
- Some hospitals will not incur management costs such as salaries for the trauma director and nurse coordinator due to the availability of existing staff or because of voluntary commitments by the medical and nursing staff.

POTENTIAL IMPACT OF NONDESIGNATION

The ramifications of not being designated as a trauma center are poorly understood because sufficient data are not yet generally available. It is reasonable, however, to assume that the annual financial impact of losing 150 to 200 trauma patients from a community hospital is far less than a gain of 300 to 400 patients by a designated trauma center.

The direct revenue implications of designation/nondesignation are outlined in Table 6.8, which reflects the existing trauma volume

Table 6.8 Designation/Nondesignation Hospital in a Northern California Hospital*

	Designation Volume (370)	Existing Volume† (122)
Revenue		
ICU/SCU	$118,000	$1,272,893
Med/Surg/Peds	169,500	827,024
Acute Rehabilitation	66,500	356,125
Ancillaries	364,500	2,525,788
Total	$718,500	$4,981,830
Average Patient Bill	$ 5,889	$ 13,464
Average Length of Stay (days)		
ICU	1.9	4.5
Med/Surg	8.8	8.0
Acute Rehab	2.9	2.5

*The above figures do not represent extended care services or readmissions to acute rehabilitation and extended care by trauma patients.

†This volume would no longer be sent to Hospital A if the hospital was not designated.

Source: EMS Systems Design, Irvine, CA

in a Northern California hospital as compared to projected volume. Other potential implications of nondesignation are listed below.

- Further reduction of emergency department visits by minor trauma or nontrauma patients
- Further reduction of medical staff specialists who may join the more dynamic trauma center staffs
- Erosion of nursing and support staff skills in the treatment of acute patients
- The necessity for an aggressive image campaign to offset the broad positive image of the trauma center
- Difficulty in recruiting emergency, intensive care, and operating room nurses and emergency physicians interested in working with trauma
- Reduction in utilization of services currently used by trauma victims affecting future certificate of need applications

It should be noted that a number of well-respected hospitals in the nation have chosen not to apply for trauma center designation as a result of competing hospital priorities, potential cost implications, or lack of a sufficient medical staff commitment. It is unlikely that such a decision will be injurious to the hospital if it has previously enjoyed a solid position in the community. In fact, in Southern California where a trauma system was implemented almost two years ago, several nontrauma hospitals have actually experienced increases in utilization of their emergency departments and certain specialty services, e.g., open heart surgery, despite predictions to the contrary.

SUMMARY

It is vitally important for hospitals to analyze the financial implications critically before choosing whether or not to become a trauma center. Some of the factors and techniques described previously may be of assistance. In order to obtain the most accurate assessment of the financial implications, the parameters listed below should be integrated into the review.

- Obtain as objective a clinical and financial review as possible from inside or outside the hospital.
- Avoid direct comparisons with other operating trauma centers
- Develop a methodology that meets the individual needs and characteristics of the reviewing hospital and service area.

Use of these parameters will enhance the ultimate result of any financial review.

REFERENCES

1. Hospital Resources for Optimal Care of the Seriously Injured. Bulletin, American College of Surgeons, February, 1980, pp. 31–33.
2. Champion, HR, Sacco, WJ, Hannan, DS, Lepper, RL, Atzinger, ES, Copes, WS, Prall, RH: Assessment of Injury Severity: The Triage Index. *Critical Care Medicine* 8:201–208, 1980.

7
THE COMMUNITY HOSPITAL AS A TRAUMA CENTER
C. Thomas Thompson, M.D.

There are so many factors that affect the development of community trauma centers that it is difficult to put into perspective the overriding needs of the severely injured patient. This is not a mere philosophical discussion, for mangled, bleeding bodies continue to arrive with regularity in, not just our university centers, but also in our community hospitals. The drive to improve trauma care in the community is born as much of necessity as of the grandiose aspiration of developing a trauma center. It is precisely because trauma patients continue to arrive at institutions without due notice that particular attention must be paid to the organization of trauma care. The university hospital, with its tightly organized services and its plethora of residents, must remain committed to the special needs of trauma patients, while the community hospital must assess its mission to see if trauma *can* become one of its commitments. Certainly, the institution that has no empty beds and whose operating suites and critical care units are stretched to capacity should not undertake the new venture of a heavy commitment to trauma.

FACTORS IN TRAUMA CARE

An analysis of some of the factors that affect the development of a community hospital's capability in trauma includes the size and location of the institution, demography of patient referral patterns, emergency department volume, admission rates, and quality of its medical staff. The needs of the indigent and the community or state commitment to meet those needs may bear heavily on the ability of an institution to be a trauma center.

Private community hospitals of insufficient size to provide full-service medical care can function as trauma centers if the commitment is there. Hospitals with 500 or more beds whose emergency departments see 50,000 or more patients annually are ideal, while small institutions often have difficulty justifying the high cost of additional 24-hour staffing.

In the private sector, an emergency department that sees 50,000 to 60,000 patients annually will admit 8,000 to 10,000 patients of whom 20 percent will be trauma victims. The number of patients with multiple or life-threatening injuries will probably account for only about 300. These are approximate figures that will differ from community to community.

Suburban hospitals are apt to be required to deal with motor vehicle injuries, while hospitals located close to the inner city generally experience higher percentages of knife-and-gun-club patients. Although the latter patient is rarely sought by the community hospital, any community trauma care plan must deal with these patients. As a result, many hospitals are not anxious for designation as a trauma center lest they become flooded with these nonpaying patients.

If a community has developed a good emergency prehospital system with effective medical control, however, the community hospital may then begin to plan for its place in that system.

STEPS IN DEVELOPING TRAUMA CARE

Assessment of Current Trauma Practice

It is essential to evaluate the current trauma patient load with some type of injury indexing. An institution with the occasional severe injury should probably opt out of the major trauma business entirely, while the hospital that currently deals with major trauma on a daily basis should look into making the commitment necessary for the highest possible level of care.

The Planning Process

Most hospitals have a mission statement that is so broad, bland, and supportive of motherhood and apple pie that it can be interchanged with that of any other hospital. Representatives of the board of directors, administration, and medical staff leadership should instead attempt to define the mission of the hospital in more pragmatic terms. Clearly, economic survival is a necessity, and the acute care, general nature of the institution must be preserved. However, areas of excellence can be defined in services such as cardiovascular disease, oncology, burns, dialysis, neonatal, etc. If a commitment to excellence in trauma care is desirable and possible, then it should be clearly articulated as an institutional mission.

Administrative Commitment

Once the trauma mission has been defined the administrative commitment to development of the necessary resources must be identified. Ultimately, this commitment must be in the best interest of the hospital in its regional setting, for no knowledgeable administrator should abandon a lucrative service for the perils of trauma no matter how loud the cry for community needs. The most difficult administrative commitment is in personnel, since hospitals are very labor intensive and all potential increases in the personnel budget must be clearly evaluated.

Task Forces

The American College of Surgeons (ACS) document, "Hospital Resources for Optimal Care of the Injured Patient,"[1] provides an excellent guideline. Task forces to review current trauma practices should be formed to define deficiencies. In this process, there will be a great amount of quibbling about the reasonable definition of optimal care. Nevertheless, task forces should report on hospital organization, special facilities, resources and capabilities, operating suite special requirements, clinical laboratory services, and programs for quality assurance. In this process evaluation of the quality of current trauma care as well as a commitment to future excellence will be established.

Medical Staff Maximally Affected

Five groups of physicians will be affected maximally by a commitment to excellence in trauma. The general surgeon, the emergency physician, the anesthesiologist, the neurosurgeon, and the orthopedist must make the heaviest commitment in terms of availability and time. An assessment of the trauma capability in each of these areas is essential. It is not enough to have a surgeon available—

he or she must be capable in trauma. The special demands of a trauma commitment may necessitate increasing considerably the staff of hospital-based physicians, including emergency physicians and anesthesiologists.

A large emergency department must have the ability to increase its staff immediately should the emergency load demand it. This need requires a plan that automatically triggers itself. Any hospital with a heavy emergency load in addition to other surgical services such as obstetrics must be certain of the immediate availability of adequate anesthetic services. The loudest outcry about the "Optimal Care" document frequently comes from institutions unwilling to meet these specialized demands.

It is the general surgeon, the orthopedist, and the neurosurgeon whose commitment must be unmistakable. The argument as to whether one can justify the cost of 24 in-house surgeons versus immediate availability of surgeons is moot. If there is a heavy trauma load and these services are committed, then all efforts should be made to support this commitment. Preferential access to the operating rooms and even the parking lot should be considered, for this is the surgical troika that can make or break the trauma service.

Medical Staff Moderately Affected

Trauma does not respect organ systems. The special services of the ophthalmologist, otolaryngologist, urologist, and other surgical specialties may be required. The services of the radiologist are invaluable and include the commitment to immediate availability of computerized axial tomography (CAT), angiography, and ultrasonography.

The major impact of the trauma commitment will be felt by the surgeons and anesthesiologists, while the rest of the medical staff will be affected secondarily. Trauma is a surgical disease and the hospital priority in this regard must be clearly understood.

Review Mechanisms

It is imperative that the review process be implemented at the outset to monitor how well the system is working. Is the continuum of care from the scene, enroute via helicopter or ambulance, in the emergency room, in the operating room, and in the critical care unit one of smooth transition? Are there mechanisms to see that the interfaces among the various members of the trauma team are identified and "turf" problems eliminated? Does the audit process address the trauma system as well as the medical care? Is there continuing leadership to upgrade any deficiencies? The final question would have to be: Do we still wish to make this great commitment to trauma in our hospital?

RESULTS OF A TRAUMA COMMITMENT

What are the anticipated results if an institution makes this heavy commitment? If the problems of penetrating trauma are great, then the economics of trauma care are dismal. In some communities, the hospital collects only 25 percent of hospital charges while the fee-for-service physicians are even less fortunate. Certainly an institution cannot survive in the knife-and-gun-club milieu unless the community assists in payment for these services. In our experience nearly 80 percent of hospital charges have been collected for the critical trauma patient brought to the hospital via helicopter or ambulance, while the fee-for-service physician charges have been reimbursed at a rate of 60 to 70 percent depending upon the specialty involved. This would imply the potential for economic viability.

The most dramatic institutional result is the marked potential for improvement in nontrauma emergency capabilities. The trauma capability makes available necessary services for the patient with a ruptured aorta or an intracranial bleed. The mobility of the diagnostic services necessary for trauma are essential ingredients for other emergencies. The *esprit de corps* generated by a team approach is a valuable spin-off.

The effects of a trauma commitment on the medical staff cannot be minimized. Heavy fatigue factors are apparent that can change the nature of recruiting for the medical staff. Sufficient numbers of hospital-based emergency physicians, anesthesiologists, and radiologists, are imperative. The hospital must encourage its private surgeons, orthopedists, and neurosurgeons to recruit young physicians qualified in trauma continually. This may require a hospital subsidy, but it does not necessarily require hospital-paid traumatologists, especially in the community setting.

The future of trauma care in the United States will depend on the commitment to excellence of our community hospitals. Trauma, which is an inescapable part of our medical heritage, is with us in increasing numbers and complexity. Neither physicians nor hospitals can shrink from this duty to our fellow man.

REFERENCE

1. Bulletin, American College of Surgeons, August, 1979.

8
THE UNIVERSITY HOSPITAL AS A LEVEL I TRAUMA CENTER
Donald D. Trunkey, M.D.

In 1976 the Task Force of the Committee on Trauma of the American College of Surgeons (ACS) published a document entitled "Optimal Hospital Resources for Care of the Seriously Injured."[1] Updated in 1979, it was retitled "Hospital Resources for Optimal Care of the Injured Patient."[2] In bringing this second document to fruition, it was recognized that there were several problems related to trauma care. The Task Force thought that in addition to optimal care there should be some impetus for education and research in the area of trauma.

To meet this need several principles were established. The primary goal of a trauma center is to provide optimal care for the injured patient. It was recognized that both community and teaching hospitals would be involved in this optimal care. It was further recognized that 90 percent of all trauma patients fall into the noncritical category. It was thought by the Task Force that this great majority of patients should be cared for by a Level III hospital, unless the patient came from a neighborhood where there was a Level I or Level II hospital. The essence of the Level III hospital was to be the commitment of the medical staff and hospital administration to provide consistent, excellent care for the less seriously injured.

The Task Force felt that the level of patient care provided by Level II and Level I hospitals should be the same. Although this is the ideal, it may not be possible in all instances since some community hospitals may have to opt for promptly available rather than in-house surgical coverage. The difference in care should be minor, and the commitment of the medical staff and hospital administration should be the same for the two levels.

In addition to excellent care, the Level I hospital has two other missions: research and education. The staffing patterns in a Level I hospital should reflect these three primary missions: excellence in patient care, research and education. In regard to patient care, the attending staff should provide the primary focus of patient care while the resident staff remains ancillary. The staffing requirements for research and education should be calculated separately from those of patient care. However, there will undoubtedly be overlap between the three areas. Ideally, the same principle will apply to nursing and others involved in the Level I center.

The staffing patterns should reflect the commitment to 24-hour, 365-day coverage, not just for the individual patient, but also for multiple patients who present at the same time. This commitment may require coordination and diversion to other trauma centers within the region or adjacent regions, especially when operating rooms or intensive care units become full.

It requires a certain volume of patients in a Level I center to maintain skills, proficiency, and cost effectiveness. In Chapter One there has been a discussion of the rationale for absolute numbers of patients based on staffing needs and their relation to Level I or Level II designation. These guidelines were developed as recommended minimal levels and should not be taken as standards, since studies have not yet shown what constitutes the lower limit for a Level I or Level II center. At San Francisco General Hospital, approximately 4,000 trauma patients are admitted annually, of whom 40 percent would qualify as Category I or II patients. This volume has not taxed the facility and its personnel beyond their limit. Other trauma centers in Houston, Dallas, and Detroit have similar or greater volumes, yet they have not been stressed beyond their limits. Undoubtedly, however, there is some finite number below which either patient care or cost effectiveness becomes important.

The Level I trauma center, in an ideal situation, should also expose residents and nurses to other types of trauma including burns, spinal cord injuries, and replantation injuries. It is not absolutely necessary that these patients be in the same hospital, but they should be exposed to such patients at some time during their training. When there are separate facilities for these entities there should be transfer agreements between the trauma center and the specialized units.

Emergency room staffing in Level I centers has produced some unique problems. On the one hand, surgical departments have tended to put unsupervised surgical residents in the emergency room to initiate the resuscitation until the trauma team arrives or the attending surgeon comes in from home. While this is not as desirable as having supervised residents or attending surgeons within the emergency area, the latter is in many instances impractical. On the other hand, some Level I centers have established emergency medicine programs and have delegated the early resuscitation to the emergency physicians and residents. Although this provides the necessary coverage, it is unacceptable in teaching hospitals in which it denies surgical residents exposure to resuscitation, which is an integral part of the care of the trauma patient.

Marriage of these two concepts is also fraught with difficulty. Attending emergency physicians involved in teaching surgical residents present special problems. Although the attending emergency physician is certainly skilled in many resuscitation techniques and the evaluation of shock, he or she is rarely qualified to teach the surgical resident sophisticated surgical skills such as emergency thoracotomy. A reasonable compromise is for the attending emergency physician to provide minute-by-minute supervision of the surgical resident with the proviso that an attending surgeon will come to the emergency room promptly when major surgical needs arise such as emergency thoracotomy or when the decisions and skills required may demand the experience of the attending general surgeon.

The same principles apply to the surgical specialists, which must provide teaching and supervision in the emergency room for their housestaff. Each Level I center has its own unique problems in meeting emergency room staffing requirements. Solutions will depend on cooperation between the various specialties, but quality patient care must remain the primary goal.

Medical control of the prehospital care system is another potential problem in the Level I center. The trauma surgeon should not abrogate the responsibility of medical control of the trauma patient to any other specialty. If other physician specialists or nurses are used for medical control of the trauma patient, trauma protocols must be developed in consultation with the trauma surgical staff to ensure optimal prehospital trauma management.

The Level I trauma center also has obligations to Level II and Level III centers. This entails provision of educational experiences for community physicians, nurses, and paraprofessionals, including provision of teaching conferences, rounds, and updates on the newest research developments. The Level I center should also serve as a tertiary care center for special problems or unique injuries such as replantation surgery, extracorporeal membrane oxygenation, and reconstructive surgery. The Level I center should additionally assume a leadership role in regional disaster planning that includes the contiguous Level II and III hospitals.

There are some unique economic issues that face the Level I center. Prior to 1966, public and teaching hospitals traditionally cared for approximately 25 percent of the population. In many instances reimbursement was provided only through local county governments or local tax districts. With the passage of Titles 18 and 19 (Medicare and Medicaid), some of these patients were shifted to community hospitals. Recently there have been major cutbacks in these government insurance programs, along with reductions in capitation funds for medical students and a gradual reduction in research secondary to inflation. All of these factors have placed constraints on university programs such as trauma. Some of the more serious problems have occurred in Level I hospitals affiliated with universities where, in some instances, transfers have actually been refused from other trauma centers. Although morally and ethically unacceptable, this is an economic reality.

The solution is obvious. Government, either local, state, or federal, must underwrite the care of the indigent patient and the illegal alien. A reasonable cost reimbursement has to be made to the Level I centers for care of these patients. Hopefully, the government and the medical community can solve this vexing issue while keeping in mind that the patient is the primary concern.

The 1979 document "Hospital Resources for Optimal Care of the Injured Patient"[2] states,

> The most significant ingredient necessary for optimal care of the trauma patient is *commitment*, both personal and institutional. For the institution, optimal care means providing capable personnel who are immediately available. It also implies using sophisticated equipment and services that are frequently expensive to purchase and maintain. It means there must be a priority of access to sophisticated laboratory and radiologic facilities as well as the operating suites and intensive care units.
>
> For the medical staff, optimal care means a commitment to the concept of prompt availability, to education, to regular audits, and to critiques, all specifically geared to excellence in trauma care. This commitment includes not only the surgical disciplines, but also involves the entire medical staff in planning and implementing optimal care for the trauma patient. At each level of service the responsibility for providing this optimal care rests inescapably with hospital boards, trustees, administrators, and medical staff. No longer can we categorize facilities without considering the degree of commitment the institution has to excellence.

The American College of Surgeons feels very strongly about these statements. How is it measured? Of prime importance in the voluntary verification process is the emergency room. The emergency room log can be used to provide the names of five to ten patients who appear to be seriously injured. Examination of the medical records of these patients will provide the necessary information regarding commitment, including response times, appropriateness of care, delays, and outcome. A comprehensive evaluation further includes conversations with the nurses in the emergency room, operating room, and intensive care units. Their observations provide an excellent source of factual, unbiased, and honest information that is useful in appraising a hospital's commitment to trauma care. Based on these two review processes one can determine whether or not the hospital has made the commitment as outlined in the American College of Surgeons document.

In summary, the Level I trauma center should be the crown jewel in a regional trauma system. The Level I institution has three missions: excellence in patient care, research, and education. Ideally the Level I center should additionally provide leadership in disaster planning, prevention, and other trauma-related problem areas.

REFERENCES

1. Bulletin, the American College of Surgeons, September, 1976.
2. Bulletin, the American College of Surgeons, August, 1979.

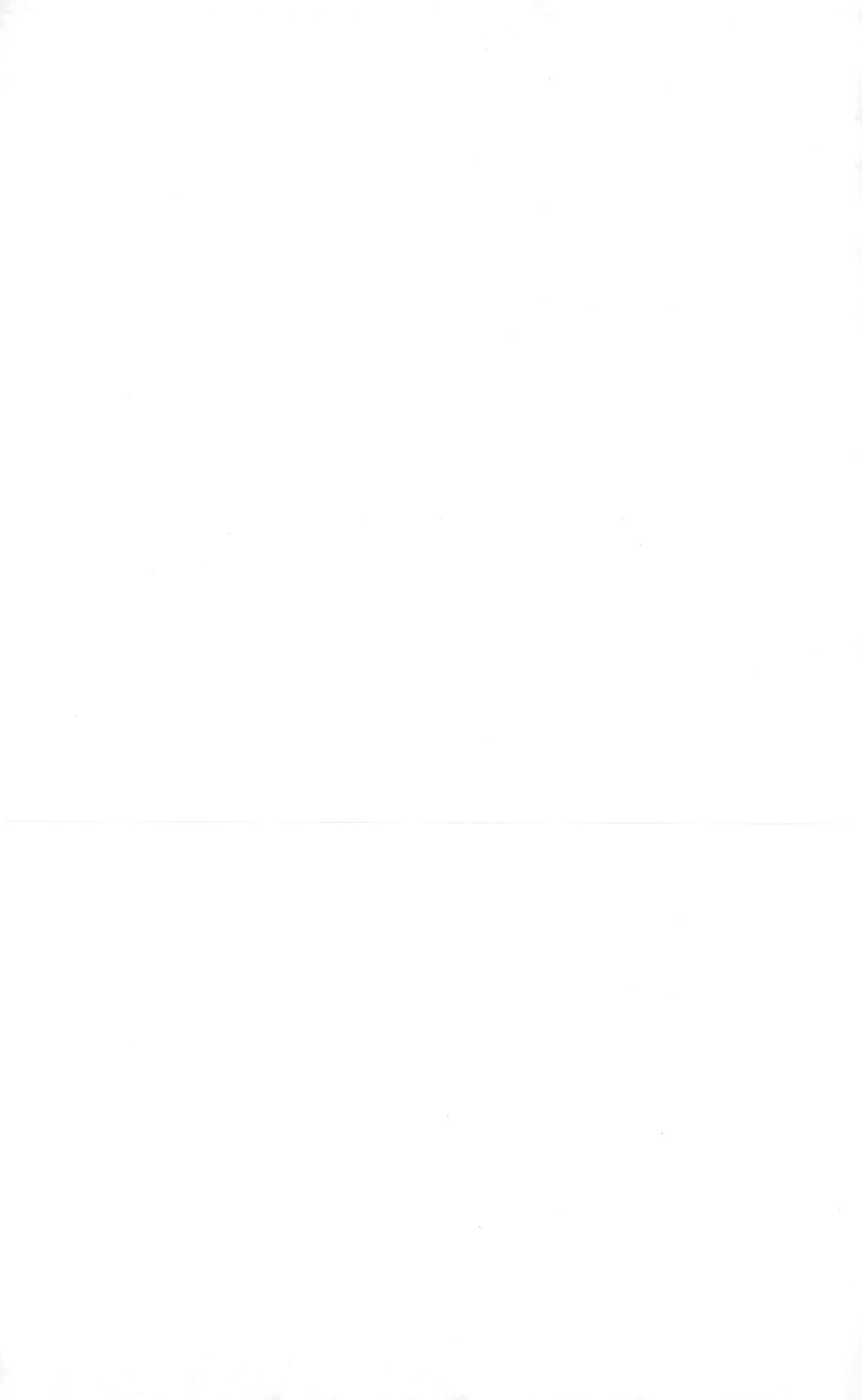

PART II
SPECIAL CLINICAL NEEDS IN TRAUMA SYSTEMS DEVELOPMENT

The selection of chapters in this section deals with the special considerations necessary to address in developing a trauma system. The subjects presented are not complete but do represent the components of specialized care that the community will expect the trauma system to provide.

Chapter 9 presents the proposed role of the trauma center emergency physician relative to hospital consultants and the emergency medical services (EMS) system in general. Dr. Charles R. McElroy advocates a prominent role for the emergency physician as the overall director of trauma care in the hospital setting. However, it would seem that the individual's qualifications are of more importance than his or her specialty background. Since there are no standards for what constitutes the person who should fill this central role in the organization of a trauma center, it should be considered unclaimed territory. The individual must be skilled in trauma management of all types, must have personal experience in the field, and must function as a part of the total organization of the hospital and medical staff. The individual should have completed a residency in order that there has been peer review of his or her skills and intellectual capabilities. Whether that person is a surgeon, emergency medicine physician, or family practitioner is of little importance.

In Chapter 10, Dr. Frank R. Lewis presents a candid and controversial discussion of the function of the paramedic in the prehospital care of the trauma patient. One cannot argue that documentation of the efficacy of any interventive therapy is a desirable goal. Rapid speed from the scene to the hospital is also crucial, but delays may be related to extrication or in securing the scene before the emergency medical technician-paramedics (EMT-Ps) can reach the patient. The physician at the hospital does not always understand the circumstances at the scene and may complain that too much time was spent by the paramedics in the field treating the patient. For example, an intravenous line can be started while the patient is still trapped in an automobile and this should not be considered inappropriate intervention.

The issue of endotracheal intubation should be faced by all emergency medical services (EMS) systems, and the esophageal obturator airway (EOA) relegated to a historical role in the development of prehospital care. Endotracheal intubation can be taught to EMT-Ps and can be done expertly in the field, as has been proven in Seattle.

The issue of the value of the military antishock trousers (MAST) suit is more difficult to resolve since it was generally introduced without preclinical trials. However, one would have to devise a very unusual and imaginative protocol to prove its efficacy. Patients would have to be randomized into two groups, and selection would have to be based on the usual criteria for MAST suit application. This would mean that for two patients with blood pressures of 40 mmHg or less, random selection would result in inflation of the MAST suit for one and not the other. It would be most difficult for a paramedic and the physician at the hospital to issue an order not to inflate when the blood pressure is zero. Also, a statistically significant number of patients would have to be studied, perhaps as many as 100. Inflation of the MAST suit not only raises blood pressure but will also often awaken a previously unconscious patient who is in shock.

The corollary to this occurs at the hospital when sudden removal of the MAST suit by inexperienced personnel may result in circulatory arrest within a few minutes in an otherwise awake, responsive patient. Therefore, any study designed to prove the efficacy of the MAST suit would by and large run into many ethical considerations as well as resistance from all levels of prehospital and inhospital personnel.

The essential issues in prehospital care in the urban setting are airway control and rapid transport. In a large territory where there is a combination of urban and suburban settings, on many occasions field stabilization may provide the additional treatment needed to deliver a more salvageable patient to the trauma center.

Once hospitals are designated as trauma centers, field triage criteria should be devised to identify those patients needing transport to a trauma center. Careful triage will ensure that the severely injured patient arrives at a trauma center. Dr. Dennis A. Wheeler presents a method for field trauma scoring and the experience of the Inland Counties of California with this system. Any triage system that is used should err on the side of overtriage in order to prevent sending a seriously injured patient to a hospital not prepared to deal with trauma.

Certain age groups and types of injuries require special care. Pediatric trauma care falls into this category. Dr. Alasdair Conn from the Maryland Institute of Emergency Medical Services Systems relates their experience with the triage of pediatric trauma patients to Johns Hopkins Hospital. Pediatric trauma patients require different fluid resuscitation, lines, and tubes, as well as different surgical instruments. Their postoperative management should be supervised by those skilled in pediatric patient management. It seems reasonable that a regional center for pediatric trauma be developed.

Dr. Lawrence H. Pitts emphasizes the importance of early intervention in the treatment of acute head injury. In the multiply injured patient, it is often not possible to obtain sophisticated studies to document intracranial bleeding. In some instances it may be necessary to do a diagnostic and therapeutic craniotomy while other procedures are underway. Dr. Pitts' aggressive approach to the neurologically injured patient is one to emulate by other trauma centers.

Microsurgery has grown enormously over the past ten years, and replantation has become a common operative procedure. Dr. Bruce M. Achauer, who has vast experience in replantation, outlines the requirements for a replantation center and presents a realistic approach to its organization.

Helicopter transport is a vital function in some EMS systems. Chapter 15 presents a series of short papers on the use of helicopter transport. The helicopter should be looked upon as an extension of the emergency department or prehospital care system that can facilitate the transport and delivery of patients to trauma centers. In any situation, the cost effectiveness of the helicopter and the potential benefits have to be carefully assessed. The potential hazards of air and on-the-ground accidents is always a consideration, particularly in congested urban areas.

This section concludes with a discussion of the U.S. Army's capabilities in emergency patient care, ground and air transport, and research in traumatic injuries. Dr. Michael R. Antopol presents the functions of the Army Medical Department in both times of peace and war.

9
THE ROLE OF THE EMERGENCY PHYSICIAN
Charles R. McElroy, M.D.

The role of a member of a health care team is determined by the specific needs of the system being constructed, the biases of the individuals involved in the design of the system, the resources available, and many other variables. This analysis will be based on my impressions of the present system of emergency care in Los Angeles County. I will discuss a reasonable and evolutionary system that uses existing facilities and personnel, adding trauma specialists and equipment only when such additions can be reasonably expected to improve (in a cost effective fashion) the care currently given.

For many reasons, Los Angeles Trauma Centers are conceived of as part of a total system of emergency care not separate physical plants with monofocal personnel. While this approach may have its drawbacks, it reflects an almost certain reality for this area.

Creation of trauma centers separate from existing emergency care centers is not only prohibitively costly but unnecessary and undesirable. The great majority of trauma victims have injuries that do not require surgical intervention. The exclusive use of trauma surgeons to direct and evaluate field care, to supervise and educate prehospital and emergency department personnel, to triage and evaluate all trauma victims, to stabilize the seriously injured, to perform the necessary emergency department diagnostic procedures, to lead the operative team in surgery, and to care for the seriously traumatized and postoperative patients in the surgical intensive care unit requires too much of individual surgeons. Several of these patient care functions can be carried out effectively by other health care personnel. The need to refine and maintain surgical skills is inherent in the concept of trauma care. Not all surgeons are equally disposed to, or capable of, performing trauma surgery. While the number of patients required may be in doubt, any system design must guarantee an adequate patient load and provide for adequate operating time for each trauma surgeon to reach as near an optimal level of performance as is practical. Therefore, it is reasonable to include participation of trauma surgeons in the design of every level of care while simultaneously insulating them from the personal involvement and responsibility for each step.

Management of trauma victims begins in the field at the earliest possible time after the injuring event. While experimentation with different systems of in-field care has led to a variety of approaches, the paramedic in our area is, and will undoubtedly remain, the backbone of field care. Design, education, monitoring, and real-time direction of paramedic activities are the provinces of emergency medicine. Emergency physicians (with appropriate consultations from cardiologists, neurosurgeons, orthopedists, pediatricians, gynecologists, and trauma surgeons) must be responsible for medical management of field operations. This responsibility involves daily contact with the administrative providers, Los Angeles City Fire, Los Angeles County Fire, private ambulance companies, and many others.

Field procedures, equipment, protocols, and performance standards must be established, integrated into the system, and monitored. Education to introduce new skills and maintain old ones is integral to the optimum performance of the system.

While the cooperation and appropriate input of trauma surgeons is imperative, to place the responsibility for this entire prehospital part of the emergency care system on trauma surgeons makes little sense. Since trauma care is but a small part of the overall prehospital operation, the generalists of prehospital care—emergency physicians—are the appropriate health care personnel to assume overall direction and medical control. Design of the trauma component, while using the expertise of trauma surgeons, must place the trauma response in perspective, creating a system of the best care for the greatest number. Inappropriate use must be minimized, unmet needs eliminated, and time and money conserved. These goals are most likely to be met when individuals with both breadth and depth of perspective are used in the design and operation of the system.

Most of the points made for patient care in the prehospital setting are relevant to patient care in the emergency department. Most trauma patients need never see a trauma surgeon. Emergency physi-

Role of the Emergency Physician

cians, trained and practiced in skills required to evaluate, to stabilize, and to treat trauma patients are the backbone of the emergency department. In a busy trauma center, as conceived for the Los Angeles County region, the seriously injured trauma victim would constitute only a small part of the daily patient load. Estimates of three to six patients a day seem reasonable given the system under consideration. Further, many of these patients would not come in prelabeled, i.e., the extent of injury would not be immediately obvious, thereby requiring quick, efficient, and reliable evaluative activities.

It is now well established that, using appropriate and reliable diagnostic techniques, emergency physicians can evaluate individuals potentially in need of trauma team consultation, stabilize them as necessary, and call the trauma surgeon when the patient has been properly prepared. The time of such consultation will vary according to the arrival times of individual patients—at times upon entry to the emergency department and at other times only after considerable evaluative and preparatory effort.

In cases of obvious severe trauma, activation of the trauma team should occur before the victim arrives in the emergency department. With appropriate field evaluation and communication, supplementation of the trauma team with necessary personnel can be anticipated. Neurosurgeons, pediatricians, orthopedists, and others who would not be primary members of the trauma team could then be notified. This activity is appropriately part of the responsibility of the emergency department physician in charge of the communications operation.

Optimally, the core trauma team includes trauma surgeons, emergency physicians, emergency nurses, and emergency trauma technicians. While it is possible to make up the trauma team using only trauma surgeons, anesthesiologists, and other personnel peripheral to the mainstream emergency department activities, inclusion of emergency physicians makes considerable administrative, organizational, educational, and patient care sense. It is, after all, the emergency physician who is most familiar with the facility, its personnnel, and the overall needs of the emergency department at any given time. Therefore, the emergency physician can best provide for optimal overall patient management.

By organizing along these lines, two specialists who must work closely together are given ample opportunity to evolve a systematic approach to trauma care that is mutually acceptable to facilitate speedy evaluation and therapy. It is imperative that a generalist be the leader of such a team. Coordination of the activities of many specialists working simultaneously on one or more patients is central to a successful resuscitative effort. Staging and scheduling of diagnostic maneuvers requires an overview of the patient's total need and must not be left to any one subspecialist. The emergency physician is the logical individual of choice to perform in this role. While such an organizational scheme requires the availability of one or more emergency physicians assigned to the trauma team, it allows for the best use of the skills of the trauma surgeon and other surgical specialists. Furthermore, it allows each of the specialists the opportunity to concentrate on the areas of patient care with which he or she is most familiar.

In summary, there are many ways to organize any system of health care delivery. In Los Angeles County we are somewhat constrained by existing facilities, personnel arrangements, and community expectations. Major modifications of existing facilities and personnel seem unlikely at a time when financial constraints are burdensome. Organization of a trauma system integrated into the already existing emergency care operation will improve patient care by providing adequate patient flow and by pairing skilled emergentologists and trauma surgeons with patients most likely to be in need of their services. Placing the emergency physician in the center of this organizational activity simply reflects the fact that emergency departments deal with a wide variety of patients. No one component should be unreasonably represented.

The fact that cardiovascular disease statistically outstrips all other life threats does not dictate that cardiologists should run emergency departments or see every patient presenting with chest pain. It does dictate that emergency personnel should be optimally familiar with emergency care of patients whose complaints may represent a cardiovascular emergency and should have immediate access to consultative support from a cardiologist when necessary. The success of emergency physicians and emergency departments in dealing with cardiovascular disease can, I think, be taken as a measure of the capability of such a system to achieve a similar success quotient for trauma victims.

Above all, reorganization of the existing system must reflect emergency physician administrative control. The emergency department is the domain of emergency medical and support personnel. All others serve best in a consultative role. Cooperative efforts to deliver optimal health care to all patients will result in the best care for the greatest number. Competition for those patients results in fragmentation of effort, administrative chaos, and weakening of the emergency system to the detriment of all.

10
PREHOSPITAL CARE: THE ROLE OF THE EMT-PARAMEDIC
Frank R. Lewis, M.D.

The data regarding paramedic field care of cardiac patients have been tacitly extended to trauma care in most areas of the country, with the assumption that field stabilization, intravenous lines, and drug treatment carry similar benefits. It is becoming increasingly clear that this assumption is not true, and that field care of trauma patients may have to be regarded differently. Patients who stand to benefit from prehospital care are those with emerging life-threatening problems. In the trauma area this usually translates into airway obstruction or exsanguinating hemorrhage. It can be argued that tracheal intubation is the safest and most definitive treatment for the former condition, yet paramedics in most areas of the country are not trained to intubate. There is virtually nothing that the paramedic can do for exsanguinating internal hemorrhage. The volume of intravenous fluids to be given during a five-to-fifteen minute ambulance ride is usually ineffective for major volume deficits, and the effects of the antishock garment appear marginally effective.

Faced with these realities, it becomes obvious that the most precious commodity is time, and the waste of it in the field by paramedics who are not providing effective treatment is probably not warranted. It seems increasingly obvious that the paramedic skills that would be beneficial for acute trauma care are very limited, and that a "load and go" philosophy should be adopted in all areas where transit times to definitive care are less than 20 to 30 minutes.

PREHOSPITAL TRAUMA CARE

The prehospital care of trauma patients has evolved during the last decade such that increasing numbers and types of intervention by paramedics are being made without demonstrated effectiveness or clinical value, without cost-benefit analysis, and without documentation of complication rates. The efficacy of prehospital care for cardiac arrest victims has been documented in several systems, with salvage rates of 3 to 20 percent. These data have been extrapolated to trauma victims, with the tacit assumption that similar intervention will have equally beneficial effects. It must be emphasized that no published data exists to support this assumption. Experience with helicopter evacuation and prehospital paramedic care in the Vietnam War was markedly better than comparable military experience in earlier conflicts. The major reason was the rapid evacuation to definitive surgical care. In Vietnam there was an average time of injury to definitive care of 65 minutes, whereas in the Korean War the comparable figure was two to four hours,[1,2] and in earlier wars was even longer.

The essential difference between the cardiac arrest victim and the trauma patient is that in the former case cessation of circulation already exists when the paramedic sees the patient. Efforts to restore circulation and ventilation are obviously necessary, because transport times to a hospital normally exceed the allowable interval before cerebral and myocardial ischemic damage become irreversible.

In trauma the physiologic situation is to a large extent the opposite. The patient starts with normal circulation and ventilation, and following a critical injury loses ground with time because of hemorrhage and/or respiratory impairment. There is little that the paramedic can do in the field to reverse the problem other than to alleviate simple airway obstruction or, ideally, insert an endotracheal tube, if he or she is one of the minority of paramedics trained in airway intubation.

The salvage of such patients largely depends on their delivery to a hospital capable of rapidly providing definitive surgical intervention. It may legitimately be argued that comprehensive field assessment and intervention, such as intravenous lines, do more harm than good because the time required for their insertion is more detrimental to the state of the severely traumatized patient than any potential benefit during a short transport to the hospital. In the cardiac arrest victim, an intravenous line is essential for the administration of resuscitative drugs. In the traumatized patient, drugs are generally not needed or useful. The only beneficial effect of an intravenous line is to give fluid for the restoration of intravascular volume. However, the size of the intravenous catheters that can be inserted in the field is so small that relatively little volume can be administered in a five-to-fifteen minute period of time.

Lest the reader think that this is an absurd point for discussion, it is useful to reference a recent paper by Gervin and Fisher.[3] The authors examined mortality in 23 patients who sustained cardiac injury. Of potentially salvageable patients, zero of seven patients transported by paramedics survived, while five of six transported by emergency medical technicians (EMTs) or by private autos survived with comparable injuries. The conclusion of the authors was that field treatment attempted by paramedics consumed time (mean = 40 minutes) that would have been better spent getting the patients to the hospital and resulted in a greater mortality. Thus, in cardiac injury paramedic intervention appeared hazardous to the patient's health.

To examine this question more closely, we need to consider the causes of death after trauma. Once these are defined, we can discuss each of them and determine the potential benefits of paramedic intervention, as well as possible detrimental effects on the trauma patient. The concept of *primum non nocere*, which is indoctrinated into physicians during their training, seems as yet not to have been a major consideration in prehospital care.

Baker et al. evaluated the causes of death in 437 patients dying during one year in San Francisco (Table 10.1).[4] Blunt and penetrating trauma accounted for nearly equal numbers of deaths, as is usual in an urban setting. In more rural areas, blunt trauma is far more common because of the preponderance of motor vehicle accidents as a cause of death.

Of the 437 patients, 232 were judged dead at the scene and were taken directly to the coroner. The primary cause of death in this group was exsanguination. Respiratory compromise due to airway obstruction or aspiration ranked second, and severe central nervous system (CNS) injury was third. Two hundred and five patients were taken to the hospital, and 32 died in the emergency department. The patients in this group generally arrived in cardiac arrest and were not resuscitatable. The primary cause of death was exsanguination.

One hundred and seventy-three patients were initially resuscitated, but 94 died in the hospital within the next 48 hours. Two principal causes of death were noted in this group: (1) irreversible CNS injury, due to either primary cerebral trauma or ischemic damage from cardiac arrest; and (2) exsanguination that could not be controlled operatively. The remaining 79 patients died after 48 hours,

Table 10.1   Causes of Death in 437 Trauma Patients

Cause	Patients Number	Percent
Brain injury	219	50.1
Heart or aortic injury	76	17.4
Hemorrhage	51	11.7
Sepsis	43	9.8
Lung injury	24	5.5
Burn	15	3.4
Liver injury	9	2.1
Total	437	100

and the majority (78%) of these were due to multiple organ failure related to sepsis or to late death from CNS injury.

If one looks at the summary data in Table 10.1, it is evident that about half the total deaths are due to CNS injury. If all the hemorrhagic lesions are grouped together, they account for about 30 percent of the total. Airway problems account for about 5 percent, and late death related to sepsis occurs in slightly over 10 percent. Let us examine each of these causes of death to see how prehospital care might impact on it.

The single most important treatment for the head injured patient (unconscious) in the prehospital setting is endotracheal intubation. Other treatment modalities do not have proven benefits and probably delay definitive neurosurgical care. When intracranial pressure is increased due to cerebral edema, mannitol may possibly be of benefit, but edema usually develops later in the course of the disease and is not a prominent problem in the first 30 to 60 minutes. Of greater importance is prompt transport of the patient to a hospital where a neurosurgeon and operating room are available, so that intracranial bleeding can be controlled and hematomas decompressed. It has been shown that improved neurosurgical outcome is directly related to the speed with which the patient is definitively treated.[5] Therefore, the principle benefit that can be offered by the prehospital care system to patients with potentially lethal head trauma is rapid transport.

Exsanguination is the second most common cause of posttraumatic death, only slightly less frequent than head injury. What can a paramedic system offer here? Basically two field treatments are potentially beneficial. The first is placement of an intravenous line and rapid administration of fluids for volume replacement. The second is application of a pneumatic antishock garment. Use of an intravenous line initially appears noncontroversial, as harm rarely results even if fluids are given to patients who do not need them. However, the time element necessary for starting intravenous lines has never been critically analyzed but almost certainly is relevant. McSwain[6] looked at the average time necessary for intravenous placement in the field in arrested patients and found it to be 12 minutes. This number seems plausible, given the adverse conditions under which the paramedics are operating. A common example is the case of a hypovolemic patient with constricted veins, decreased cardiac output and arterial pressure who is in a poorly lit area and possibly a moving ambulance. One wonders, in fact, what the overall success rate is in starting intravenous lines under such circumstances. It would not be surprising to find rates as low as 50 percent, but to the best of my knowledge the problem has not been studied.

Assuming that the 12-minute average time is representative of other systems, what does it tell us? Obviously, the first conclusion is that it is foolish to start an intravenous line if the transport time to a hospital is less than 12 minutes. Under such circumstances the patient could be in an emergency room with the full range of services available before the intravenous line could be started. In fact, this circumstance applies to most ambulance runs in the urban setting!

What if the transport times are longer? To answer this we need to consider the rate of bleeding necessary to cause exsanguination. First, consider the case in which bleeding is at such a rate that the patient will exsanguinate in 10 to 15 minutes. Such patients will rarely survive in any system. By the time an ambulance is called, responds, and transports the patient to a hospital, the total elapsed time will usually be greater than 15 to 20 minutes. Hence, the patient will have arrested prior to hospital arrival. In such a circumstance it is clear that attempts to start an intravenous line are misguided. The time wasted in such an attempt is far too precious and should be spent moving the patient. In addition, the rate of bleeding in such cases will be at least 150 ml per minute, far in excess of the rate of replacement possible through the usual 18-gauge venous cannula. Thus, even if an intravenous line is started it will not be possible to approach a replacement rate necessary to stabilize the patient.

At the other end of the spectrum is the patient who is bleeding slowly and would not exsanguinate for at least one to two hours. It is evident that in the usual urban setting the patient will reach the hospital well before a critical volume deficit exists. Thus, in this patient as well, starting an intravenous line serves no useful purpose and only delays transport.

What of the third case—moderate rates of bleeding that would cause exsanguination in 15 to 60 minutes? Given the physiologic fact that patients must lose 40 to 50 percent of their blood volume before cardiac arrest occurs, it is clear that the rate of bleeding in such cases must be generally in the range of 30 to 100 ml per minute. At the upper end of this range, it is clear that the rate of intravenous replacement, which even with manual pumping rarely exceeds 50 ml per minute, will be slower than the rate of bleeding. It is therefore impossible that the cost in time of starting the intravenous can be made up by subsequent volume infusion. At the lower end of the scale, the rate of replacement becomes comparable to the rate of bleeding; thus for the first time the potential benefit exceeds the cost in time. The point at which this occurs obviously cannot be specified precisely, but would appear to be near 30 to 40 minutes. It therefore appears that the only situation in which delay in the field to start an intravenous line might be justified is when transport time to the hospital will exceed 30 to 40 minutes. Such a circumstance is quite rare in the urban setting, but it is commonly seen in rural environments. It would therefore appear that, in general, the use of intravenous therapy in most cities is contraindicated.

Obviously, if a "scoop and run" philosophy is adopted and attempts to start an intravenous line are made only after the ambulance is moving, the above analysis does not apply, as no delay in transport results. Our practical observation, as well as the observation of most paramedics and physicians with whom we have discussed this issue, is that paramedics will generally resist such a policy. They clearly know how difficult it is to start an intravenous line in a moving ambulance and, therefore, tend to make every attempt to get it in at the scene, not realizing how much time is consumed in the effort. It is imperative that this problem in medical control be recognized and dealt with if trauma salvage is to be improved.

In the previously cited article by McSwain, the potential adverse impact of the delay in starting an intravenous line was documented. The report looked at outcome in 100 patients who had a field cardiac arrest. The survival rate was compared to two groups; those in whom an intravenous line was attempted (whether successful or not), and those in whom no attempt was made. Although the numbers are not large, the survival rate was 14 percent if no intravenous line was attempted and only 5 percent if it was attempted. Thus it appears that patient outcome was significantly worsened by the intravenous therapy attempt and was directly related to the extra time taken in the field. This study is unique in that it is one of the first in the literature that attempts to look quantitatively at the value of paramedic service. Additional studies in a variety of locations, carefully controlled for cause of death, are badly needed.

Role of the EMT-Paramedic

The second modality that is potentially beneficial in the hypovolemic trauma patient is the pneumatic antishock garment. It was introduced in Vietnam, felt to be generally of value, and is now a standard item in most paramedic jurisdictions. Nevertheless, at the risk of being thought an iconoclast, I must point out that there has never been a study done in any scientifically acceptable way that proves it is of value. One can state with certainty now that the generally accepted explanation of why the pneumatic antishock garment raises blood pressure is false. It was previously thought to generate an autotransfusion of 500 to 1000 ml of blood from the legs and pelvis into the upper body circulation. Recent studies[7] have shown that the actual transfused volume is of the order of 200 ml—hardly enough to have a significant impact on patient survival. Further, the mechanism by which it raises blood pressure is simply an increase in peripheral resistance. Nevertheless, this may be a useful maneuver, as available cardiac output is redirected to the most critical areas of the body.

There are, however, three potentially negative effects to be considered. The first is the time necessary to place the garment and inflate it. Although no published data are available, this is probably 5 to 10 minutes on the average. For the same reasons given previously for intravenous lines, use of the antishock garment is not justifiable if done at the scene. The second potential negative effect is that raising blood pressure in a hypotensive patient by increasing afterload may accelerate the rate of bleeding and actually hasten the time at which a critical volume loss will be reached. The third negative effect is that the upper portion of the antishock garment restricts expansion of the lower ribs. In the patient with concomitant respiratory impairment, this may worsen an already critical respiratory state.

For the above reasons, it is not possible to conclude *a priori* that the pneumatic antishock garment is beneficial in trauma. Its effects are complex and only a carefully done prospective study will answer the question. If the actual benefits of the pneumatic antishock garment are marginal or nonexistent, then its high cost cannot be justified.

The third cause of death in trauma patients, which accounts for approximately 5 percent of the total, is respiratory failure. This problem usually results from airway obstruction due either to aspiration or coma, but it may also result from open pneumothorax, tension pneumothorax, or flail chest. Paramedics are taught to use a variety of airway maintenance devices; however, evidence of their effectiveness is again lacking. It is noteworthy that the most widely accepted of these devices, the esophageal obturator airway (EOA), has recently been shown in the first objective prospective study available to produce adequate ventilation of patients only 25 percent of the time.[8] If these results are duplicated in other studies, it is obvious that a better method must be found.

The most effective and safest method of airway maintenance is the endotracheal tube. Paradoxically, a minority of paramedics are trained in its use. This is no doubt because the skill is difficult to acquire and maintain, and easier methods have previously been thought adequate. In the future it seems likely that this skill should receive greater emphasis, perhaps at the expense of other training for which little patient benefit can be shown.

SUMMARY

The value of paramedic treatment in the prehospital care of trauma patients appears to be minimal. Available literature suggests that field intervention attempted by paramedics may increase mortality rather than decrease it, principally because of the additional time consumed. Deaths resulting from head injury and exsanguination, which account for 80 percent of the total, are not effectively treatable by paramedics in the field unless transport time to definitive care exceeds 30 minutes. In contrast, the short transport times usually found in the urban environment argue against paramedic intervention, as it is likely to be more harmful than beneficial. The pneumatic antishock garment, while widely accepted and used, in fact has not been shown to be effective, and studies of its value are clearly needed.

Of the remaining deaths in the field, respiratory compromise is the principle cause, and endotracheal intubation is the most effective treatment. Paramedic training in this skill should probably become universal. Although not yet proven, there is suggestive evidence that the widely used esophageal obturator airway is ineffective in a large percentage of patients and should be abandoned.

The preceding observations document that prehospital care has evolved in ways that are not in the best interests of trauma patients and that the time is overdue when paramedic care must be subjected to the same kind of scrutiny as other areas of medicine. The field has grown exponentially in the last decade due to large infusions of federal and other funding with the underlying belief that more is always better and that what is good for cardiac patients will also be good for trauma victims. Both of these assumptions are clearly false, and it is time that prehospital trauma care is placed on a more solid scientific base.

REFERENCES

1. Byerly, WG, Pendse, PD: War surgery in a forward surgical hospital in Vietnam. *Military Med.* 136:221, 1971.
2. Trunkey, DD: The value of trauma centers. Bulletin of the American College of Surgeons, 67:5–7, 1982.
3. Gervin, AS, Fischer, RP: The importance of prompt transport in salvage of patients with penetrating heart wounds. *J. Trauma* 22:443, 1982.
4. Bauer, CC, Oppenheimer, L, Stephens, B, Lewis, FR, Trunkey, DD: Epidemiology of trauma deaths. *Amer. J. Surg.* 140:144, 1980.
5. Seelig, JM, Becker, DP, Miller, JD, Greenberg, RP, Ward, JD, Choi, SC: Traumatic subdural hematoma: Major mortality reduction in comatose patients treated within four hours. *New Eng. J. Med.* 304:1511, 1981.
6. McSwain, GR, Garrison, WB, Artz, CP: Evaluation of resuscitation from cardiopulmonary arrest by paramedics. *Ann. Emerg. Med.* 9:341, 1980.
7. Bivins, HG, Knopp, R. Iernan, CT, dos Santos, PAL, Kallsen, G: Blood volume displacement with inflation of antishock trousers. *Ann. Emerg. Med.* 11:409, 1982.
8. Smith, JP, Bodai, BI, Ward, RE: Effectiveness of the esophageal obturator airway in cardiopulmonary resuscitation. Presented at the 42nd Annual Meeting of the American Association for the Surgery of Trauma, September 10, 1982 (*J. Trauma*) 33:23–28, 1983.

11
MECHANISMS OF PREHOSPITAL IDENTIFICATION OF TRAUMA PATIENTS
Dennis A. Wheeler, M.D.
Bridget Simone, M.P.H.

In the Inland Counties Emergency Medical Services (EMS) region of California, the death rate from motor vehicle accidents is substantially higher than elsewhere in California and in the nation as a whole. This problem stimulated the local EMS agency to place priority on the role of the EMS system in trauma. The local medical community recognized the need for a structured program to improve care of the severely injured patient. Therefore, in 1979 the concept of a system of designated trauma centers to which victims could be directed to ensure rapid, appropriate care was endorsed.

The Inland Counties Emergency Medical Authority (ICEMA) was charged with the responsibility of managing the designation process. In conjunction with the medical community, ICEMA was to develop an effective method of providing triage for victims that would ensure the timely transport of severely injured persons to the most appropriate hospital, while not diverting an undue number of patients who could appropriately be managed by the hospital nearest to the scene of the accident.

Fundamental to this process was the need to identify lethal injury in the field. There were three reasons for this.

- Implementation of the trauma system field response only when it was necessary for good patient management
- The preference of trauma center designees not to be overloaded with unnecessary high volumes of minor trauma
- Implementation of a method for field identification and triage which demonstrated that overall patient destination patterns

would not be substantially changed, and further, that bypass of the closest hospital would predictably occur only in that small percentage of patients who would benefit from immediate hospital intervention.

In 1979 ICEMA was fortunate to be asked to review the work of Dr. Howard Champion with respect to field-testing its use as a triage tool. The work was of great interest because it appeared to have the potential to meet our criteria for a field triage methodology, i.e., it was quick, simple, and reliable. Speed was needed so that decisions could be made under field conditions in a matter of seconds to avoid delaying transport to a trauma center. Simplicity was required so that the data could be obtained reliably, predictably, and reproducibly by hospital personnel (in our area, primarily by paramedics). Reliability meant that the method should not be liable to subjective bias on the part of the reporter and that it could be scientifically and statistically validated to correlate with lethality. Using Dr. Champion's trauma score, a triage methodology was developed that appeared to meet the above criteria.

The trauma score is based on variables from the three body systems that are primarily involved in early death from trauma: central nervous, cardiovascular, and respiratory. Weighted values are assigned to each system to obtain a trauma score. The values vary from 1 (the worst prognosis) to 16 (the best prognosis and maximum score). Figure 11.1 demonstrates how the score is compilated and Table 11.1 correlates the score with the probability of survival.

We found that the data needed to secure a patient's trauma score can be obtained from a trained prehospital provider in a very short time, and the score can be rapidly computed by the base station physician. The question remains, however—is this trauma score in itself an adequate tool on which to base the decision to direct a patient to a trauma center? Our experience is that it is not.

The trauma score is a reliable and good measure of physiologic distress at the time it is assessed (assuming the assessment is accurate), and that is all. It does not measure or predict deterioration or the period of time over which deterioration might occur. It cannot predict occult, lethal injuries, which are numerous and common.

Since implementation of our trauma system on January 2, 1980, we have developed a triage rule to determine

- Trauma Score of 12 or less → transport to a trauma center
- Glasgow Coma Scale (GCS) of 10 or less → transport to a trauma center

Figure 11.1 Compilation of the Trauma Score.

		Rate	Codes	Score
A. Respiratory Rate		10–24	4	
Number of respirations in 15		25–35	3	
seconds; multiply by four		>35	2	
		<10	1	
		0	0	A.____
B. Respiratory Effort		Normal	1	
Retractive—Use of accessory muscles or intercoastal retraction		Retractive	0	B.____
C. Systolic Blood Pressure		≥90	4	
Systolic cuff pressure—either arm		70–89	3	
auscultate or palpate		50–69	2	
		<50	1	
No carotid pulse		0	0	C.____
D. Capillary Refill				
Normal—Forehead or lip mucosa color refill in 2 seconds		Normal	2	
		Delayed	1	
Delayed—More than 2 seconds capillary refill		None	0	D.____
None—No capillary refill		Total		
		GCS Points	Score	
E. Glasgow Coma Scale		14–15	5	
1. Eye Opening		11–13	4	
Spontaneous	____4	8–10	3	
To Voice	____3	5–7	2	
To Pain	____2	3–4	1	E.____
None	____1			
2. Verbal Response				
Oriented	____5			
Confused	____4			
Inappropriate words	____3			
Incomprehensible sounds	____2			
None	____1			
3. Motor Response				
Obeys commands	____6			
Purposeful movements (pain)	____5			
Withdraw (pain)	____4			
Flexion (pain)	____3			
Extension (pain)	____2			
None	____1	TRAUMA SCORE		

Total GCS Point (1 + 2 + 3) _____   (Total Points A + B + C + D + E)

Table 11.1 Probability of Survival (P_s) by Trauma Score

Trauma Score	P_s (Washington)
16	1.00
15	1.00
14	.99
13	.97
12	.91
11	.77
10	.66
9	.46
8	.28
7	.15
6	.07
5	.03
4	.01
3	.00
2	.00
1	.00

- Trauma victim with a score higher than either of the above, but with either of the following mitigating circumstances: (1) mechanism of injury (ejected from vehicle, high-speed auto accident, vehicle versus pedestrian, fall greater than 20 feet, etc.), (2) anatomic derangement (penetrating wound to the head, neck, thorax, pelvis, etc.), → transport to a trauma center

Figure 11.2 presents the decision algorithm used by the base hospital physician in determining the trauma patient's destination in accordance with the triage rule. It will be noted that the trauma victim in full arrest is directed to the nearest facility. This is an arguable point, but the decision in our system was researched locally because of the long distances between trauma centers.

It would be idle to suggest that we have not encountered problems in implementation of a field triage methodology. The most serious of these was the initial tendency to go by the numbers and only use the trauma score in making the triage decision. This has been overcome by enhancing the role of the GCS and emphasizing the evaluation of mechanisms of injury. Further problems have been encountered with phraseology, for example, "shallow respirations." Paramedics frequently report shallow respirations in persons who are breathing normally. We find the term relatively meaningless and in need of change. Preferable terminology characterizing respiratory distress, such as "retractive breathing," is being considered. Pediatric patients present problems in that the GCS cannot be readily obtained, especially in infants. We find that paramedics do not use

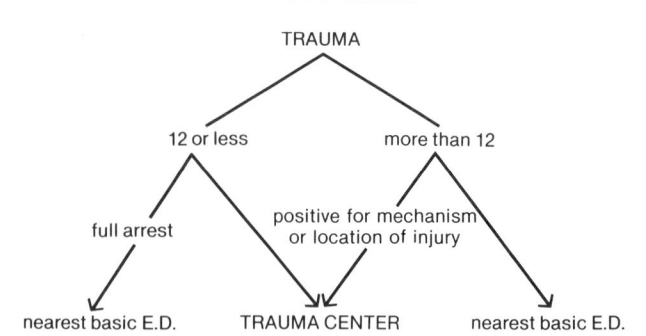

Figure 11.2   The Triage Rule Used by the Base Station Physician to Determine Trauma Patient Destination.

```
                    TRAUMA
                   /      \
            12 or less   more than 12
             /    \       /      \
            /      \  positive for mechanism
       full arrest  \  or location of injury  \
           ↓         ↓↓                        ↓
     nearest basic E.D.  TRAUMA CENTER   nearest basic E.D.
```

pediatric cuffs well nor do they uniformly carry them in the field. We have found that the GCS is not being assessed as accurately and uniformly as initially anticipated. Within busy emergency departments where frequent one-on-one debriefing can be done, it has been shown that emergency medical technicians (EMTs), nurses, and physicians score patients similarly and accurately. In our system, paramedics are given a brief instruction in GCS scoring and then actually perform it clinically on their own in the field, on an occasional basis. More attention needs to be focused on the development and maintenance of skills in this regard.

At least as interesting as the problems associated with trauma triage have been the unforeseen benefits. Clearly, the most rewarding unanticipated benefit has been the region-wide focus of attention on rapid assessment and transport. Unnecessary and time-consuming assessment and treatment in the field had long been a deleterious factor in the care of the severely traumatized in our system. Since no formal mechanism existed to identify those types of patients who benefit from *limiting* the paramedic activity in the field, we were grossly ineffective in enforcing such behavior. By doing so with the triage rule, wherein all secondary assessment of the critical patient is done en route, we can now limit such activity. By eliminating untoward field delay in rapidly deteriorating trauma victims we may have done as much to influence favorable outcomes with respect to trauma in our region as the designation and activation of specialty trauma centers has done.

12
PEDIATRIC TRAUMA: THE BALTIMORE EXPERIENCE
Alasdair Conn, M.D.

My pediatric colleagues kept referring to the fact that pediatrics brings with it certain special and unique problems of patient management, and is more than the adult traumatized patient in miniature. For this reason, a Pediatric Trauma Center situated at the Johns Hopkins Hospital has gradually evolved within Maryland.

In the early days, the main Shock Trauma Unit in Baltimore had an open-ended admission policy. It would accept all traumatized patients regardless of age, and, in particular, it did not want to split up the family in terms of a multicasualty situation. However, the incorporation of a pediatric trauma load within the adult population did not appear to be cost effective. Additionally, it put extremely high stress on the surgical and nursing staffs.

The number of pediatric trauma cases in Baltimore is relatively low. The existing data show that the city has approximately 1,400 pediatric trauma cases a year. This figure also represents the maximum patient load that can be managed by the present physical limitations of the hospital. Approximately 80 percent of the med-evacs involve children less than biological age 14. As a criteria, we use a biological age such that a large 11-year-old can easily be managed in an adult trauma center and a small 15-year-old can be best managed in a pediatric center.

In 1977, Professor Haller of Johns Hopkins Hospital approached the Maryland Institute of Emergency Medical Services Systems (MIEMSS) stating that he was interested in expanding his role as a pediatric surgeon. He stressed that trauma was the number one cause of death of children and that he had a pediatric intensive care unit (ICU) that was not being used to its appropriate capacity. This seemed the ideal trade-off. We were being overloaded in the main unit and could easily transfer patients to the Johns Hopkins Hospital. At the same time this allowed us to concentrate on our goal of acute management of adult trauma. Professor Haller's program had the expertise in terms of pediatric nurses, pediatric surgeons, and intensivists in his own pediatric ICU.

There are several advantages to the segregation of pediatric trauma:

1. The cost associated with obtaining the necessary instrumentation (which includes not only surgical instruments, but also ventilators, intravenous drip sets, etc.) and monitoring equipment would be approximately $100,000 a year. When one is already dealing with adult trauma, this is not cost effective.
2. On the few occasions when the pediatric center does go on fly-by or is temporarily closed, the psychological stresses associated with management of trauma in the child are different. These patients are often referred for additional counseling.
3. Management of the pediatric patient cases are difficult in terms of drug dosages, types of medications, and problems of intensive care. Obviously, it is advantageous to use existing resources fully.
4. Isolation of pediatric trauma also brings an isolation in terms of magnitude of the problem. Johns Hopkins currently manages approximately 400 patients a year. They are transferred by surface and helicopter transport. The magnitude of this problem became evident, and statistics can be provided from this single institution in terms of prevention. For example, safety seat legislation was presented before the legislature in Annapolis in the last session.
5. The management of certain types of injury is unique in the pediatric situation. Concentration of this specialized subgroup enables expertise, for example, in conservative management of the splenic injuries (this has now spread to adult populations) and also the management of pediatric closed head injuries.
6. Effective use of support such as the Ronald McDonald House and special expertise in terms of social work has created a more effective delivery of service to the citizens.
7. Private funding from certain citizen action groups at both the local and national level has been more effective.
8. Many general surgeons and emergency department physicians are more amenable to direct referral of the pediatric patient to a pediatric center (rather than to an existing trauma center), if not

for their acute emergency care, then certainly for their intensive care and follow-up.
9. Children function well in an environment in which there are other children. Hopefully, this will also decrease the stress level of the patients themselves.

13
AN AGGRESSIVE APPROACH TO THE NEUROLOGICALLY INJURED PATIENT
Lawrence H. Pitts, M.D.

The role of neurosurgery in the management of trauma is clear and vital. In a variety of studies that describe the mortality from trauma, head injury accounts for about half of the trauma deaths. That fact has been reflected by the experience in Orange County as well as at San Francisco General Hospital. The head injury population spans a broad spectrum of injury severity, from patients who suffer a mortal injury at the time of impact to those patients who almost certainly will have a good outcome unless there is a management accident that would worsen the outcome. Although it is difficult to prove unequivocally that any particular current head injury treatment has improved outcome, there is general agreement that the aggressive management of the neurologically injured patient does reduce mortality and diminish morbidity.

In recognition of the importance of neurosurgical involvement in trauma care, the American College of Surgeons has recommended that neurosurgical departments are necessary for Level I and II trauma centers, along with general and orthopedic surgery and anesthesia. For Level I trauma centers, the inhouse presence of general surgeons and neurosurgeons is deemed essential. Neurosurgeons must be available promptly in Level II and III trauma centers. However, because of the prevalence of craniocerebral trauma and the relatively limited number of neurosurgeons, neurosurgical department chiefs are encouraged to train trauma physicians in the immediate evaluation and treatment of severe head injury until a neurosurgeon arrives.

The emergency treatment of head injury is almost identical to that of the general trauma patient. It is essential that resuscitation not be delayed because attention is misdirected to documentation of obvious neurologic abnormalities such as pupillary dilatation or motor posturing. At the roadside, field management includes airway management, control of hemorrhage, and, depending on the transfer time, reestablishment of the circulating volume by placement of intravenous lines. In urban areas with short transport times, I support minimal field stabilization and rapid transport to receiving centers where definitive resuscitation can be carried out. In more rural areas where long transfer times are a rule, somewhat more time will have to be spent at the roadside trying to stabilize the patient prior to beginning the ambulance run.

In the emergency room setting, prompt attention must be given to ventilation and circulation. These are profoundly important for the head injury patient. About 30 percent of head injury patients have an arterial PO_2 below 60 mmHg, and some 50 percent of these patients have a PO_2 below 80 mmHg. It is imperative that an airway be established. Even if the comatose patient appears to have adequate ventilation, it is good practice to intubate comatose patients routinely to protect the airway. Additionally, patients hyperventilated to arterial CO_2 pressures of 25 to 30 mmHg will have acutely lower intracranial pressure. Hyperventilation is continued until the patient shows neurological improvement or intracranial pressure monitoring is established and shows that hyperventilation is unnecessary.

Head injury alone does not produce shock. If shock is present, it must be assumed to be from hypovolemia secondary to blood loss from some other organ injury. It is well documented that up to five units of blood can be sequestered in a hemothorax, in the abdomen with the rupture of a visceral organ, in the retroperitoneal area secondary to pelvic fractures or vascular injuries, and in the thighs from femoral fractures. Therefore, in resuscitation of head injury patients in shock, large volumes of fluid should be used to restore the blood pressure, and appropriate diagnostic tests initiated to locate the probable source of hemorrhage. An exception to this rule of head injury is terminal brain failure, which may not produce shock. Medullary death removes neurally mediated peripheral vascular tone, reduces peripheral vascular resistance, and increases peripheral blood pooling. This terminal medullary failure is invariably accompanied by loss of medullary function, including loss of respiration, cough, and gag reflexes. Resuscitation is usually only transiently successful; the patient rapidly dies despite support.

There is an overwhelming influence of shock on outcome from

head injury. Patients with coma-producing head injury at our institution have a 50-percent mortality when shock is not present. The combination of coma-producing head injury plus shock is attended by a precipitous rise in mortality to 80 percent.

Multiple system trauma is common in patients with head injury. Forty percent of our patients with severe head injury also have significant injury to one or more other organ systems. There is a 15-to-20-percent incidence of severe facial, chest, abdominal, or extremity injuries alone or in combination. The incidence of shock rises steadily with injuries to additional organ systems outside the central nervous system. Head injury plus one other major injury gives a 45-percent incidence of shock and a 48-percent mortality at San Francisco General Hospital. As additional injuries are added, the incidence of shock rises. At our institution, those few patients with severe head injury plus significant facial, chest, abdominal, and extremity injuries had an 80-percent incidence of shock and all died.

Thus, initial therapy is designed to restore rapidly and maintain blood pressure. If adequate perfusion can be readily established with prompt resuscitation, further studies are appropriate to evaluate treatable central nervous system lesions. These are best evaluated with computerized axial tomography (CAT) scanning. If the blood pressure cannot be maintained after initial resuscitation, the patient undergoes rapid evaluation for other sources of blood loss, including chest x-ray and peritoneal dialysis to look for evidence of visceral bleeding. If a hemothorax is found, a chest tube is placed and subsequent operative management depends on the rate of bleeding from the chest. If peritoneal dialysis is positive, the patient is taken directly to the operating room. In these circumstances, the neurosurgeon has adequate information regarding intracranial pathology. Therefore, if the patient was comatose in the emergency room, temporal and frontal burr holes are placed bilaterally to detect the presence of extracerebral hematomas. If none are found, a catheter is placed in the right frontal horn and 5 cc of air and 2 cc of conray are injected. An anteroposterior skull x ray is obtained on the operating room table while thoracic or abdominal surgery proceeds. This contrast ventriculogram allows the neurosurgeon to determine midline shifts that might warrant burr holes or a craniotomy. In addition, the intraventricular catheter allows the neurosurgeon to detect elevated intracranial pressure in the operating room and treat it appropriately with hyperosmolar agents and hyperventilation. If the patient can be stabilized after surgery, he or she is usually taken for a CAT scan immediately following surgery. In those few instances where an operable intracerebral hematoma is found, this patient would return to the operating room for a craniotomy and hematoma evacuation.

If a patient is only lethargic on admission, but peritoneal dialysis is positive and immediate abdominal exploration is indicated, the neurosurgeon will generally place a twist-drill burr hole at the right coronal suture for placement of an intraventricular catheter at that time. A contrast ventriculogram is carried out as described previously; further operative intervention will be decided depending on the x rays. If a patient has an obvious head injury but is awake following resuscitation, we sometimes use what I call "observation under anesthesia," which is tricky at best. This presumes that an abdominal exploration can be done in a short period of time so that the patient can be awakened quickly and more detailed neurological evaluations can be done sequentially.

Fortunately, most of the anesthetic agents used do not cause pupillary changes. Progressive pupillary dilatation can usually be detected even in anesthetized patients. If prolonged thoracic, abdominal, or orthopedic procedures are necessary, the recommended treatment is to place an intraventricular catheter for monitoring intracranial pressure during surgery.

THE NEUROLOGICAL EVALUATION

An accurate baseline neurological evaluation is important in allowing subsequent observers to determine a patient's improvement or deterioration. A very simple standardized examination can be done in 60 to 90 seconds and will provide ample information to determine the patient's current neurologic status and a baseline against which to compare future observations and possible changes.

The Glasgow Coma Scale (GCS) is an excellent measure of level of consciousness. Evaluation of eye-opening response, best motor response, and best verbal response allows an accurate way to determine a patient's level of consciousness and is vastly superior to such subjective terms as "lethargic," "stuporous," or "obtunded." The motor response scale (flaccid, extensor posturing, flexor posturing, normal flexion, localizing, and following commands) provides a basis for determining the quality of motor response and should be used in lieu of such phrases as "purposeful," or "semi-purposeful" motor movements. These terms quite often have different meanings for different observers.

Although errors can be made in obtaining a proper GCS, in general, the interobserver variability is minimal with these observations. In our estimation, the GCS is the most reliable and easiest measure of hemispheric function currently available to us. Its use should be strongly encouraged throughout all phases of head injury care, spanning from the prehospital field evaluation through the emergency room and into the intensive care and acute care hospital settings.

Other neurologic signs that should be elicited include pupillary response to light as a measure of upper brainstem function, extraocular movements with either the doll's eye maneuver,* or ice water caloric testing. Medullary function is most easily evaluated by observing ventilatory patterns and testing for cough and gag reflexes. Cough and gag reflexes should be done only in the emergency room setting, since pharyngeal or tracheal stimulation might produce vomiting with subsequent aspiration and airway compromise in the head injury patient. This simple scheme of GCS and upper and lower brainstem evaluation provides an excellent basis on which to base diagnostic and therapeutic courses.

If a patient is comatose, we initially administer our "coma cocktail," consisting of 50 cc of 50 percent dextrose in water to treat for the occasional hypoglycemic coma, 0.4mg of naloxone for possible narcotic overdose, and 100 mg of thiamine for occasional alterations in consciousness produced by Wernicke's encephalopathy seen in alcoholic patients. Patients with obvious evidence of brainstem compromise may go directly to the operating room for burr hole exploration. In some institutions, patients undergo CAT scanning before any intracranial intervention. While we cannot strongly disagree with this approach, there is an obligatory 15 minutes or longer spent in obtaining a CAT scan. If there is brainstem compression, this period may be critical. While diagnostic burr hole placement will not detect intracerebral hematomas, they almost always will detect subdural and epidural hematomas. Removal by craniotomy will most rapidly decompress the brainstem.

The liberal use of mannitol in the emergency room and operating room settings has a place in the management of head injury patients. Our rule for the use of mannitol is to "use it when you are going somewhere," i.e., when the patient is being taken for immediate CAT scanning, or to the operating room for burr hole placement. We never use mannitol when the decision has been made to observe the patient. Mannitol can diminish brain volume and obscure progressive hematoma formation, which can then be manifested by rapid neurologic deterioration at a time when additional mannitol and hyperventilation may not be beneficial. The usual initial mannitol dose is 1.5 gm/kg. Although we have not seen any complications with this initial

---

*Caution! Head turning can be done safely only after negative cervical spine x rays are obtained.

osmotic load, theoretically it could cause congestive heart failure in a patient with marginal cardiac status.

At our institution, corticosteroids are no longer used in the management of acute head injury. A study recently completed at our facility showed absolutely no beneficial effect on outcome from head injury. Two hundred and seventy-four patients were prospectively and randomly placed into three treatment regimes (placebo, low dose, and megadose regimens of dexamethasone).

The emergency management scheme that is currently followed dictates emergency CAT scanning or possible diagnostic burr holes for comatose patients with evidence of head injury, either by history or external evidence of injury, and signs of brain stem compression (coma, third nerve palsies, unilateral posturing). Brainstem compression should be relieved as rapidly as possible, although this group of patients taken straight to the operating room is not large.

Patients who present with focal signs but without obvious brainstem compression, require an intracranial study, usually CAT scanning. Angiography was previously the procedure of choice, but a CAT scan gives vastly superior information in the trauma patient. In a few institutions without a CAT scanner, digital venous angiography may provide a satisfactory intracranial study. However, in my judgment, virtually no institution should attempt to manage severe head injury without the immediate availability of a CAT scanner at all hours of the day and night.

The most difficult group of head injury patients to assess is that group of patients without focal neurologic deficits, typically patients who are lethargic or confused, many of whom are intoxicated. Alcoholic intoxication adds a particularly dangerous aspect to the evaluation of the head injury patient. In virtually all large series of head injury patients, there were some errors in diagnosis and treatment resulting from interpreting an altered mental status as being alcoholic intoxication when, in fact, the patient had a focal intracranial pathology, such as a subdural hematoma. While all drunk patients with a head bump cannot undergo CAT scanning, an attempt to minimize the patient's risk should be undertaken. At the time of initial evaluation, a decision should be made as to how quickly a given patient should show improvement. This decision is based on the patient's degree of lethargy or confusion as well as on the severity of head injury as assessed by history or external evidence of injury. If the patient has not shown clear-cut signs of improvement over an interval ranging from one-half hour to several hours, a CAT scan should be done to rule out an intracranial mass lesion. It should be stressed that this approach is particularly important in the elderly patient with a head injury. Such patients can harbor a slowly expanding intracranial hematoma without focal signs and will deteriorate abruptly and herniate in a short period of time. Thus, this protocol allows for a more liberal use of CAT scanning of lethargic, elderly head injury patients in the hope of detecting an intracranial hematoma before such herniation occurs.

CONCLUSION

It is clear that medical and surgical therapy cannot lessen the brain damage incurred at the time of impact, i.e., the primary injury. This can be ameliorated only by more uniform use of protective devices, such as seatbelts, shoulder harnesses, and helmets; by elimination of handguns; by a more uniform observance of speed laws; and by other preventive measures.

The challenge to physicians treating head injury patients is to detect and reverse those insults that produce secondary injuries to the brain, including shock, hypoxia, intracranial mass lesions, and cerebral ischemia caused by brain swelling. The early therapy outlined in this chapter addresses the most crucial sources of secondary brain injury. A pressing sense of urgency to diagnose potentially treatable lesions, such as hematomas, will further improve outcome statistics in patients with severe head injury. There is no question that patients do better when their hematomas are removed at a time when they are only lethargic, as opposed to removal of a hematoma after herniation.

The advent of excellent emergency medical services with rapid transport times and the availability of CAT scanning should allow physicians to intervene in patients earlier than in the past. It is by judicious application of the sophisticated medical system available to us that we will be able to minimize the devastating effects of central nervous system trauma and optimize patient outcome after severe head injury.

REFERENCES

1. Jennett, B, Teasdale, G, Braakman, R, Minderhoud, J, Heiden, J, Kurze, T: Prognosis of patients with severe head injury. *Neurosurgery* 4:283, 1979.
2. Braakman, R, Gelpke, J, Habbema, JDF, Maas, AIR, Minderhoud, JM: Systematic selection of prognostic features in patients with severe head injury. *Neurosurgery* 6:362, 1980.

3. Miller, JD, Butterworth, JF, Gudeman, SK, Faulkner, JE, Choi, SC, Selhorst, JB, Harbison, JW, Lutz, HA: Further experience in the management of severe head injury. *J Neurosurg* 54:289, 1981.

4. Clifton, GL, Grossman, RG, Makala, ME, Miner, ME, Handel, S, Sadhu, V: Neurological course and correlated computerized tomography findings after severe head injury. *J Neurosurg* 52:611, 1980.

5. Greenberg, RP, Becker, DP, Miller, JD, Mayer, DJ: Evaluation of brain function in severe human head trauma with multimodality evoked potentials. *J Neurosurgery* 47:163, 1977.

6. Gennarelli, TA, Spielman, GM, Langfitt, TW, Gildenberg, PL, Harrington, T, Jane, JA, Miller, JD, Pitts, LA: The influence of the type of intracranial lesion on outcome from severe head injury: A multicenter study using a new classification system. *J Neurosurg* 56:26, 1982.

7. Becker, DP, Miller, JD, Ward, JD, Greenberg, RP, Young, HF, Sakalas, R: The outcome from severe head injury with early diagnosis and intensive management. *J Neurosurg* 47:491, 1977.

8. Bowers, SA, Marshall, LF: Outcome in 200 consecutive cases of severe head injury treated in San Diego County: A prospective analysis. *Neurosurgery* 6:237, 1980.

9. Pitts, LH and Martin, N.: Head Injuries. Symposium on Trauma. *Surg Clin of NA* (62):47, February, 1982.

14
THE ORGANIZATION OF CARE FOR THE PATIENT WITH A SEVERED LIMB
Bruce M. Achauer, M.D.

Although the first limb replantation was performed in 1962,[1,2] only within the past five years has this become a standard of care available throughout the country. The most significant recent development was the evolution of microsurgical techniques. The first successful replantation using microsurgical techniques was performed in 1965.[3] Large series began to appear in the literature in the late 1970s.[4,5] Today, anyone with an amputated limb fully expects to go to a hospital and have it replaced with virtually normal function. In a recent suit, the author gave expert testimony that replantation of an avulsed index finger at the proximal interphalangeal level was contraindicated. The jury still awarded a judgment to the plaintiff because he was not offered the choice of replantation.

There seem to be no clear-cut definition or defined role for a replantation center. This chapter will attempt to define a "center" as opposed to a "service" as well as discuss the advantages and disadvantages of centralization. Information was gathered from a nationwide questionnaire sent to all members of the American Society for Surgery of the Hand (not an official society survey; this was done by the author and does not reflect any policy of the society). Other organizations involved in extremity trauma were also consulted, including the American College of Surgeons Committee on Trauma, the American Academy of Orthopedic Surgery, and the New York City Emergency Medical Service.

WHAT IS A REPLANTATION CENTER?

One approach to a definition would be to list the ideal components and call institutions meeting these requirements "centers" and those having only the basic essentials a "service." Elements of a replantation center include the following.

Surgeon

A fully trained microvascular surgeon who is a competent hand surgeon is essential. His or her background may be in plastic, orthopedic, or general surgery. At least two such surgeons would be necessary to provide 24-hour-a-day, 7-day-a-week service. Therefore, at least two staff level replantation surgeons should be available at a "center" although a solo surgeon could provide replantation "service" when he or she was available. The surgeon will also need assistants. A variety of sources are possible, including residents and fellows, other staff physicians, or nurses and physicians' assistants trained in microsurgery.

Operating Microscope

A two-man operating microscope designed especially for hand surgery is required.

Experienced Operating Room Personnel

The care of the special instruments and the microscope must be handled by trained people.

Postoperative Care

The first few hours following surgery are crucial, as many early failures can be salvaged if recognized early. Experienced intensive care unit nurses and sophisticated monitoring equipment are required. Patients should not be transferred for "postoperative care" as has occurred at our center.

Therapy and Rehabilitation

Return of useful function should be the goal. Careful integration of therapy is essential. The therapists should be very familiar with the rehabilitation of the replanted limb.

Laboratory

A microsurgery laboratory is essential for training and research and useful for maintaining competence. Availability of a laboratory would be another distinguishing feature between a "center" and a "service."

SURVEY RESULTS

Respondents

One hundred and forty-five hand surgeons replied to the 500 questionnaires mailed. The respondents were heavily weighted toward replantation surgeons. Eighty-three stated they were involved in replantation. Nine respondents stated there was a single staff-level surgeon involved in replantation, but they felt they worked in a center. Two did occasional replantations but did not feel that they worked in a center. The most common situations were two staff surgeons (20 responders) and three staff surgeons (25 responders). There are two large centers in the country: Baltimore and Louisville. Almost all respondents had residents or fellows also involved (totaling at least 325 trainees). Interestingly, two centers use "microassistants," i.e., physicians' assistants or nurses trained to assist in microsurgery.

Location

Most centers were well spaced from one another. Examples include Denver, 600 miles to the next center; New Mexico, 500 miles; and Louisville, 400 miles. A 200-mile separation was most common and was the case for Atlanta, Memphis, Baltimore, and Durham (Duke). Several major cities have more than one center: San Francisco, six; Chicago, five; and Boston, four.

Case Load

How many cases a year are required to maintain competence and to be called a center? Most say there is such a level, but it has not been defined. In the survey, the most interesting division of responses was between those doing replantation and those not doing replantation. Twelve out of fourteen nonreplantation surgeons felt more than 20 cases a year were necessary to maintain competence.

Thirty-one of fifty-five replantation surgeons who answered the question felt that fewer than 20 were sufficient.

Should There Be a Regional or National Communication Network?

One nonreplantation surgeon felt that "more surgeons trained in this technique will be coming into the market place and will dissolve the need for centers in a sea of quality care." The Microsurgery Committee of the American Society for Surgery of the Hand conducted a survey in 1976. Fifty-four out of seventy-five respondents felt regionalization was desirable for replantation centers.

ADVANTAGES OF REPLANTATION CENTERS

1. Referring physicians can be assured of 24-hour-a-day, 7-day-a-week service, which might save time compared to trying to locate a solo practitioner.
2. With more than one staff-level surgeon available, a second case or an extremely complex case can be accommodated. In the survey, most centers could perform and have performed simultaneous replantations.
3. Results are said to be improved with increased experience and continued practice, which is probably the crucial point. If results are better, the center concept should be encouraged.
4. Improved selection of cases became apparent with experience. Surgeons became more adept at determining who will really benefit from replantation and who should not be offered replantation. Experienced surgeons can back this decision in court if necessary; those with little experience are taking a greater risk, and may also waste a great deal of effort.
5. There is a more efficient use of time, personnel, and equipment with experience. If this is true, these advantages add up to more cost-effective procedures.
6. Better postoperative monitoring will occur. The crucial first few postoperative hours require careful monitoring for salvage of early failures. Few nurses are capable of doing this, unless they are experienced and trained.
7. Therapists can become proficient in the special needs of replantation patients.
8. Equipment can be better utilized. Operating microscopes and microinstruments are expensive. They are cost-effective if used frequently.

DISADVANTAGES OF REPLANTATION CENTERS

1. Patients may have to travel substantial distances. Although this is usually possible, it may become impractical. For example, a farmer in Montana might benefit from replantation but would not be willing to travel several hundred miles away to have the procedure done. Also, therapy and rehabilitation are needed for weeks and months postoperatively. The patient cannot remain 200 miles from home for this amount of time. An additional problem with widely spaced centers is ischemia time for amputated parts containing significant amounts of muscle tissue. Every minute saved in getting these parts revascularized results in higher survival rates.
2. Smaller organizations are more efficient than large ones. This is a theoretical argument.
3. Establishing centers will upset some people. This is a major obstacle in organizing any health care system.
4. Replantation centers may not be necessary.

WHAT HAVE OTHERS DONE?

Various regional authorities throughout the country are establishing trauma centers. Often replantation is a part of this program. In the Maryland system, one hospital is assigned extremity injuries, while pediatric and burn patients go to different facilities, and the rest go to the shock trauma unit.

In Orange County, California, one center having both a burn center and a replantation center was designated a Level I Trauma Center, while other hospitals in the system not having these facilities were designated Level II Trauma Centers.

The Emergency Medical Service of New York City has written standards for replantation centers. These include: (1) at least 20 clinical microvascular cases a year (not all have to be replantations); (2) a microsurgical laboratory; and (3) at least two staff-level microsurgeons. This document also includes approximately 50 pages of general requirements for the hospital. An annual report is also required for continued designation as a replantation center.

The American College of Surgeons Committee on Trauma is preparing a report on replantation centers. The American Academy of Orthopedic Surgery is in the process of preparing a roster of replantation centers.

CONCLUSIONS

Any amputated part should be considered for replantation. With proper cooling, ischemia times of eight hours are no problem. Therefore, patients can be routed to replantation centers 200 to 600 miles away (amputations involving a large amount of muscle are exceptions).

Most surgeons actively involved in replantation feel "centers" are preferable to "services," not only for efficient health care delivery, but also for obtaining the best results. Regional health care authorities have begun designating and defining replantation centers. At least one organization is preparing a roster of replantation centers throughout the country. A roster of centers that contains specific facts (i.e., the number of surgeons, number of cases, and laboratory and training facilities) would be very useful for emergency physicians as well as promote better communication among centers. It is important that this list be as compehensive as possible, therefore, more than one specialty organization should be involved in its preparation.

REFERENCES

1. Malt, R, McKhann, D: Replantation of severed arms. *JAMA* 189:114, 1962.
2. Chen, C, Chien, Y: Salvage of the forearm following complete traumatic amputation. *Chinese Med J* 82:632, 1963.
3. Komatsu, S, Tamai, S: Successful replantation of a completely cut-off thumb. *Plast Reconstr Surg* 42:374, 1968.
4. Biemer, E, Duspiva, H: Early experiences in organizing and running a replantation service. *Brit J Plast Surg* 31:9, 1978.
5. Weiland, H, Villarreal, R: Replantation of digits and hands: Analysis of surgical techniques and functional results in 71 patients with 86 replantations. *J Hand Surg* 2:1, 1977.

15
HELICOPTER TRANSPORT SYSTEMS
Alasdair Conn, M.D.
Nina Merrill

The helicopter originally appeared as an attack aircraft in World War II. The original design was specifically for the movement of troops and later was adapted for evacuation of the injured. The original helicopters traveled at slow speeds and carried up to two patients in litters. Following World War II, helicopter use gradually moved into the civilian setting, with an ever-increasing number of states now having sophisticated helicopter transport systems.

The purpose of the helicopter is to provide rapid transport over long distances for critically ill and injured patients. This rapid transport allows the patient to be moved to a hospital where a sophisticated level of care can be instituted rapidly. In the urban setting, the helicopter can provide rapid transport to the appropriate facility bypassing congested highways and thoroughfares. In the rural and suburban settings, the helicopter can transport patients over long distances for proper care at a tertiary care center. It will also allow for extrication from rugged terrain or areas inaccessible to conventional transport.

In addition to the advantage of rapid patient transport, helicopter transport systems also allow expertly trained personnel to be transported to the victim so that resuscitation begins immediately. Rapid transport without proper initial therapy would be of no great advantage to the patient. Personnel traveling in helicopters must be highly trained to care for patients in the air as well as on the ground. Several recent reports have described the need to coordinate the efforts of medical personnel and helicopter pilots.[1-6]

Air-hospital transfer of patients to centers that provide a sophisticated level of care is also an important advantage. For example, the transport of a neonate with respiratory distress from a small hospital to a neonatal center can be greatly facilitated by the use of a helicopter.

The primary disadvantage of helicopter use is the cost, which must be paid by the patient or a third-party system. Constant evaluation of the cost-benefit ratio must be done in order to avoid overutilization of services. Although the needless transport of patients will creep into any organized helicopter system, properly done audits will help control this abuse. In many cases, overland transport of patients is still more effective, less expensive, and, in some ways, safer than helicopter transport.

Although the risks to personnel of life-endangering situations in helicopter transport is small when compared to the number of flights made, fatal helicopter accidents have occurred. A recent helicopter crash in Southern California resulted in the deaths of the pilot, copilot, and all medical personnel, as well as that of the neonatal patient.

HELICOPTER TRANSPORT: URBAN AREAS
Nina Merrill

Life Flight of Southern California services a large urban area of the Los Angeles Basin and surrounding counties. These boundaries also include rural and suburban areas. In this operating area, there are over 200 hospitals and 300 responding units. This hospital-based helicopter program operates within an emergency medical services (EMS) system that strictly dictates the responding agency and the receiving facility. Under these circumstances it would seem difficult for a hospital-based helicopter program to integrate into this system.

Despite the size and scope of the system covered, uniformly high standards are not always achieved. For example, not every hospital is qualified to handle every patient problem. This is particularly true for the multiply injured patient, the burn patient, and the patient who needs replantation. Because time can be so crucial to a successful outcome, Life Flight may be the only method of transport for these patients from one hospital to another. Unfortunately, Life Flight of Southern California is not yet accepted within the EMS prehospital care system.

Hospital-based helicopter programs are looked on by prehospital care providers as potential competitors intruding into territories where patients will be diverted from local hospitals. It must be stressed that a hospital-based helicopter program in any environment is not a replacement for an effective EMS network. The purpose of using the helicopter is to augment the existing system and to provide services to the hospitals and communities that need this resource.

Safety is the primary concern in the operation of a helicopter system in an urban setting. The skies of the Los Angeles Basin are congested, and all constraints placed on helicopters are there for reasons of safety. California has a unique requirement: All helipads must be licensed by the State Department of Transportation. This process is no less a bureaucratic adventure than application for a Certificate of Need, and is, therefore, costly and time consuming. Therefore, 60 percent of Life Flight's helicopter runs do not involve the use of licensed helipads. Our alternative is the designation of safe emergency landing zones for pickup and delivery of patients. Hospital-based programs in the state of California are currently working with the Department of Transportation to encourage them to recognize air/medical evacuation systems and to incorporate our needs for safe landing zones within their regulations.

The Federal Aviation Agency has divided the densely populated areas of the United States into terminal control areas (TCAs), and the

Los Angeles Basin is one of the busiest. While in the TCA, the helicopter must remain in constant contact with one of the more than 25 controlling air towers. For example, on a flight from Memorial Hospital in the city of Long Beach to Daniel Freeman Hospital in the city of Englewood (a ground distance of 20 miles and a seven-minute flight), the helicopter must communicate with more than four air traffic control towers. Over the years, we have developed an excellent relationship with the air traffic controllers and they are very quick to respond to our needs for immediate access.

Unlike rural areas, urban helicopters must adhere to designated routes and flight patterns. At certain times of the year, weather is a real problem. Not only must we be concerned about the weather at the pickup and destination points but also about conditions enroute. One tends to think of fog in San Francisco, but Los Angeles has its fair share.

Communications during transport are an essential feature in order for the helicopter crew to communicate with the various hospital and EMS providers. These communication systems are in addition to the required aircraft radios necessary for tower communication.

The hospital-based helicopter program must be funded and demonstrate a favorable cost-benefit ratio. A complete discussion of cost factors is not within the intent of this chapter, however, at a minimum, it must be stated that helicopter programs are not cheap. Successful integration of a helicopter transport program into the total emergency services system is primarily dependent on the commitment of the sponsoring facility. One hospital in the southern California area, for example, considered a helicopter program as a tremendous asset to the community and to its own public image. The hospital administration viewed this program as a way of making a public statement about its commitment to ensure quality medical care to the community. Additionally, it was perceived as a way to aid their physicians in providing medical care for patients who were not within their usual geographic area. It has enabled this hospital to expand other hospital services. Our helicopter works with the perinatal outreach program, the neonatal intensive care unit, the hyperbaric unit, and a nearby children's hospital.

Given the successful experience that is now a part of the history of Life Flight of Southern California, we believe that the future of hospital-based helicopter transport systems is closely tied to the expansion and future of any EMS system.

HELICOPTER TRANSPORT: THE MARYLAND EXPERIENCE
Alasdair Conn, M.D.

The experience in Maryland has been with the utilization of the state police helicopter system rather than a hospital-based program. There were many problems associated with this decision, and the system has often been criticized for the lack of experience and expertise of the medic observers.

The initial program began in 1969 with the use of two Bell-Jet Rangers of the Maryland State Police Aviation Division in cooperation with the developing Shock Trauma Unit at the University of Maryland Hospital. The Bell-Jet Rangers were modified so they could contain two litter patients and fly directly to the institute. Additionally, a parking lot adjacent to the hospital was modified to become a heliport.

The experience was controversial, to say the least. Although the police had EMS radios and police radios in their vehicles and could be in direct contact with the state police at the scene of accidents, considerable controversy existed as to whether the patient should be taken by land to the nearest hospital or by air to the Shock Trauma Unit, which, in many cases, was many miles away.

The initial service, therefore, concentrated on interhospital transports, particularly transferring patients from peripheral hospitals to the University Center. At the same time the amount of equipment carried on the helicopters gradually increased to include oxygen, airways, and military antishock trousers (MAST). The State Police medics began taking additional training and were licensed as emergency medical technicians (EMTs). With the demand for trauma care increasing and with a vigorous public relations campaign underway, other types of transfers besides trauma were piggybacked onto the existing communications and transfer system.

With the certification of the medics as EMTs and close cooperation at the local level, some of our critics' doubts began to dissipate. The governor himself strongly supported the system after an experience with a personal friend who was injured and ultimately cared for at University Hospital. With time, demands for direct scene pickups increased. Credibility was also given to the program when the Shock Trauma Unit staff became intimately involved in the training, certification, and testing of all emergency medical technicians-paramedics (EMT-Ps) in the state. Obviously, as personnel were educated in the techniques of advanced life support, they were also educated to the advantages of the treatment of burn patients in burn units; premature babies in neonatal centers; spinal cord injury patients in neurocenters; and of course, trauma patients in the Shock Trauma Unit.

The Maryland State Police has increased its operation and now has approximately ten helicopters. At this time these units are in service 24 hours a day. In 1982, a fifth operation became operational in western Maryland. Helicopters are staffed by first-responder-trained pilots and medics who have had paramedic training. They are licensed state troopers who function in two capacities. Approximately 40 percent of Helicopter I's air time is devoted to state police activities (traffic surveillance and crime suppression) and 60 percent of its time doing med-evacs. The medic observer is trained as a paramedic and licensed by the State Board of Medical Examiners of Maryland in exactly the same way as all other paramedics of the state.

There are approximately 30 medic observers in the state of Maryland. Because of the configuration of the state and the relatively short transport times (flying time is usually less than 20 minutes from the scene to the trauma center), we infrequently use physicians or flight nurses. The only exception is with the transport of neonates. There is a special cadre of advanced life support nurses trained in intubation and insertion of chest tubes in the neonate. When requested by the referring physician, these nurses are immediately available from one of the neonatal centers. In approximately 80 percent of the transports, the medic observer is able to manage the case. For the remaining 20 percent, a nurse and, occasionally, a physician are required.

Over the last 10 years we have completed approximately 15,000 transports. In terms of patient transfers, we have averaged a 22-percent-a-year increase that shows no signs of diminishing. Further efforts will be made to expand the skill level of paramedics in helicopters to include central venous line insertion and use of the McSwain Dart catheter. These innovations are anticipated within the next two years.

Utilization of the state police system in this way has, despite the growing pains, several advantages.

1. As a state resource, they are directly budgeted from the state and not built into hospital rates.
2. The fact that they are not hospital based means less antagonism among other hospitals that feel such patients are stolen from their catchment area.
3. The aircraft is maintained by the Maryland State Police. Medical liability and control of all equipment are overseen by the Maryland Institute for Emergency Medical Services Systems.

REFERENCES

1. Duke, JH, Clarke, WP: A university-staffed, private hospital-based air transport service. *Arch. Surg.* 116:703, 1981.
2. Cooper, MA, Klippel, AP, Seymour, JA: A hospital-based helicopter service: Will it fly? *Ann. Emerg. Med.* 9:451, 1980.
3. Mackenzie, CF, Shin, B, Fisher, R, Cowley, RA: Two-year mortality in 760 patients transported by helicopter direct from the road accident scene. *Amer. Surgeon* 12:101, 1979.
4. Cleveland, HC, Bigelow, DB, Drácon, D, Dusty, F: A civilian air emergency service: A report of its development, technical aspects, and experience. *J. Trauma* 16:452, 1976.
5. Felix, WR: Metropolitan aeromedical service: State of the Art. *J. Trauma* 16:873, 1976.
6. Jessen, K, Hagelsten, JO: S-61 helicopter as a mobile intensive care unit. *Aerospace Med.*:1071, September, 1974.

16
ADVANCES IN THE MILITARY MANAGEMENT OF MASS CASUALTIES
Colonel Michael R. Antopol, M.D.

The United States Army Medical Department is charged with the responsibility of providing care to our soldiers and their family members, both in peace and in war. The very nature of this responsibility demands readiness of both personnel and equipment. As a result, the army is continually updating its equipment and constantly training large numbers of medical personnel for both the active army and the reserves. On an average day in 1981, army hospitals admitted 1,089 patients, had 7,339 inpatient beds occupied, saw 61,068 clinic patients, and delivered 115 babies. Our soldiers and their equipment must be able to perform in any of a number of geographic and climatic conditions from the desert to the arctic, from the seacoast to the mountains, in jungles, or in temperate climates. We must have a readily available armamentarium of hospitals, equipment, and personnel that can be immediately utilized. A reservoir of experienced personnel exists in the active army, but the majority of our mobilization resources are in the reserve and the National Guard. Equipment available to support our soldiers is in standard sets and kits that can be transported or prepositioned. Personnel can pick up equipment either at a port of embarkation or at its final destination.

Military sick and injured are not different from civilian sick and injured. Over the years, we have responded to a large number of domestic and international disasters. Medical units of the U.S. Army have supported humanitarian relief efforts at the Teton Dam disaster, the Mt. St. Helens volcanic erruption, the Italian earthquake, the Cheyenne, Wyoming, tornado, the Bolivian air disaster, the Johnstown flood, and the Guatemala earthquake as well as twenty-five other calamities since 1975. Army resources have consistently been utilized for humanitarian efforts over the years, because we have both medical personnel and equipment that are readily available and mobile. The key in both civilian and military emergencies is to be able to get the medical team with its equipment and the patient together in the most expeditious manner.

Medical support for the individual soldier begins at the unit level. The first organic medical support is at the battalion, where emergency medical care is rendered. Battalions are grouped together and form brigades, which in turn are grouped together to form divisions. The second level of medical support is at the division, where initial medical, resuscitative surgical, and limited psychiatric treatment are available. The grouping of two or more divisions forms a corps, which is the largest ground force that contains all the necessary elements required for sustained tactical operations. The third level of medical support is at this level, and not only resuscitative but also definitive hospital care is available. The first three levels consist principally of mobile units, including hospitals. The communications zone (COMMZ) is the rear of the theater of operations and contains the fourth level of medical support where resuscitative and restorative hospital care is available. The zone of interior (ZI) is that part of the United States not included in the theater of operations and contains the fifth level of medical support. The fourth and fifth levels are characterized by large fixed hospitals that provide definitive medical care.

In designing medical support units and defining their functions, we must always provide for immediate resuscitation and rapid evacuation to a point where the injured soldier will receive adequate treatment. Treatment is provided at a series of levels, from the simplest to the most complex. Since treatment may be carried out by multiple providers at multiple facilities, there must be an integrated system designed to provide continuity of care. The battlefield is anything but static, and, therefore, our units and equipment must be mobile. The type and frequency of casualties demand a flexibility of the composition and assignment of our medical units. As a result, we can tailor our supplements either as to size or composition, depending on the need.

At the unit level, each line battalion has a medical platoon. This is the most forward medical facility where triage, emergency treatment, and disposition are carried out. This platoon has three functions that are provided by different elements: (1) the aide men assigned to render emergency medical care at the company level;

(2) the evacuation element, which collects and moves casualties to the unit aid station; (3) the air station itself where further emergency treatment is available.

The second level of medical support is provided at the division. Here there is a greater concentration of medical manpower, equipment, and expertise. A medical battalion is organic to and supports each division. Initial resuscitative medical and surgical treatment can be provided. The battalion has a psychiatrist and a mental health section with limited psychiatric treatment capability. There is a preventive medicine section, optometry and dental sections, medical resupply, and, in the air assault division, an organic air ambulance platoon. The battalion supplies forward medical companies, which have treatment and initial resuscitative capability to each of the brigades within the division. The company has an ambulance platoon for the evacuation of casualties from the battalion aid station to the medical company. Each brigade surgeon, a physician, provides technical supervision of the physician assistant at the battalion level. The medical support company in the division rear has a patient-holding capability (160 cots) for short periods (up to 96 hours) of care.

It is at the corps levels that the majority of combat medical support exists. The corps is the largest ground force that contains all the combat, combat support, and combat service support groups required for sustained tactical operations. The corps is made up of three to five army divisions and is the basic unit employing combined arms services. It is tailored for the environment and the accomplishment of specific missions. The corps controls the hospitals that are attached and support the army divisions as necessary. Generally, there are four types of hospitals available. The first is the new mobile army surgical hospital (MASH), which is a 60-bed facility (Table 16.1). It is 100-percent mobile and has four operating rooms; two of which can operate on a 24-hour basis and two of which operate on a 12-hour basis. The second is a combat support hospital (CSH), a 200-bed facility providing resuscitative surgery and medical treatment for critically ill patients. It has four operating rooms and is 35-percent mobile with its own organic transportation. The evacuation hospital (EVAC) is a 400-bed hospital that provides resuscitative surgical and medical treatment for the critically injured or ill patients and then prepares them for further evacuation. It is the most complete medical treatment facility in support of the corps and can provide specialty care for ophthalmologic, neurosurgical, neurologic, otorhinolaryngological, oral surgery, cardiothoracic, maxillofacial, psychiatric, and severely burned patients. This hospital, which is usually under tentage and has a 400-bed capability, can divide into

Table 16.1   Mobile Army Surgical Hospital (MASH).

Mission:
To provide resuscitative surgery and medical treatment necessary to prepare critically injured and wounded patients for further evacuation

Capabilities
Mobility: 100% with organic transportation
60 beds (20 preoperative/40 postoperative)
Four operating rooms (ORs)
24-hour continuous operation:
  All four ORs on 12-hour basis
  Two of the four ORs on 24-hour basis
Two central material services (CMS)
ORs and CMS housed in MUST expandable shelters. Remainder of hospital under conventional tentage (or TEMPER tents or 2:1/3:1 shelters).
Air transportable in USAF aircraft (C-130, C-141, C-5A).
TOE equipment 168,000 pounds (11,050 cubic feet)
Non-TOE equipment 62,300 pounds (3,550 cubic feet)

three 100-bed hospitalization units, each of which can operate in a different location. It may be utilized in a corps area to augment other combat zone hospitals, but it is usually assigned to provide treatment of the indigenous population and/or displaced persons or as a temporary hospital facility in the communications zone.

Other hospitals in our inventory that are utilized outside the corps area are the station hospital, which may be a 200-, 300-, or 500-bed hospital, a convalescent center, and a 1,000-bed general hospital. In addition, any hospital can be augmented by special medical teams; either of a surgical, medical, or support nature. Each corps is allocated one mobile army surgical hospital, one combat support hospital, and two evacuation hospitals per division. This combination will provide 20 operating rooms and 1,060 hospital beds per division.

A recent reappraisal of our needs has led us to once again bring the MASH into our inventory. As has been previously noted, these hospitals are 100-percent mobile and provide resuscitative surgery and medical treatment necessary to prepare critically injured and wounded patients for further evacuation. It is personnel and technology intensive and specifically designed to treat large numbers of traumatic injuries. The hospital has 60 beds, 20 of which are preoperative and 40 are postoperative. Patients are evacuated to other supporting hospitals as soon as they are stable. There are four operating rooms, all of which can operate on a 12-hour basis and two of the operating rooms can operate on a 24-hour basis. There are two central material supply services (CMS). Both the operating rooms and the CMSs are housed in medical unit, self-containing, transportable

(MUST) expandable tentage. The entire hospital, as are all of our combat zone hospitals, is air transportable in U.S. Air Force aircraft: C-130, C-141, or C-5A. The hospital itself has approximately 230,000 pounds of equipment occupying about 14,600 cubic feet. All component parts of the hospital can be moved by organic ground transportation or by the new UH-60A helicopter. The hospital staff is composed of 230 individuals, 66 of whom are officers and 164 are enlisted. There are 16 medical corps officers and one dental corps officer. Including the commander, there are eight general surgeons, three orthopedic surgeons, one thoracic surgeon, one oral surgeon, two anesthesiologists, and two emergency physicians. There are 41 army nurse corps officers, including one nurse administrator, seven nurse anesthetists, nine operating room nurses, and 24 medical-surgical nurses. Of the 164 enlisted men, there are 25 operating room/central material supply technicians, 20 patient care specialists (the military equivalent of licensed vocational nurses), 43 medical specialists or aid men, four orthopedic specialists, and five x-ray specialists. It is this type of highly flexible and mobile surgical and nursing intense facility that can be rapidly utilized not only in combat but also in a mass casualty situation with a preponderance of trauma victims. It can be rapidly moved from area to area without discontinuing care by escheloning two separate components. The MASH can care for a large number of patients and prepare them for rapid evacuation following stabilization. Its capabilities can be easily supplemented with additional surgical or nursing teams.

There are a number of shelter alternatives that our combat hospitals can utilize. Our combat support hospitals are currently housed in MUST shelters. These are large, inflatable shelters that provide the best and most controlled environment in which our personnel and our patients currently can be housed. Functional under all climatic conditions, they are transportable, well equipped, self-contained, and can be set up in a relatively short period of time. In Vietnam, however, several drawbacks were recognized. Though they are 100-percent transportable, they are bulky, require continued maintenance, and are vulnerable. Highly trained maintenance personnel are required to keep the gas turbine generators operational. Additionally, the generators are noisy, require large quantities of fuel, and are expensive to maintain.

In a rapidly moving combat situation in a temperate climate, lighter shelter alternatives would be necessary. In some instances, the old army general purpose medium tent (GP Medium) has been utilized for this purpose. The army is currently testing a new type of tent called TEMPER (Tent, Expandable, Modular, Personnel). It is light weight and has an aluminum frame, over which 100-percent polyester fire retardant fabric is placed. It can be used either individually or joined together to form a large composite tent. The TEMPER tent has doorways, windows, floors, and a liner that may be added to tailor it to more extreme climatic conditions. It is planned to use this tent in combination with other types of shelters to provide a highly mobile and versatile lightweight facility.

Another alternative is the expandable shelter. Currently, there are small expandable shelters as components of MUST in which the operating rooms, CMS, x ray, pharmacy, and laboratory are housed. These shelters expand from a single box, in which the component equipment is stored, to a box approximately twice the original size. While the operating rooms are excellent and well equipped, they are small and not well suited to a mass casualty situation. The air force and the army are currently working on prototypes of larger expandable shelters. These are called ISO shelters (international standardization organization). The shelters are normally the size of the trailer on a tractor trailer and can be expanded either to twice or three times normal size. They will give us the ability to house a large emergency room complex or an operating room with the capability for multiple patients. It is hoped that by integrating these shelters in the configuration of the combat zone hospitals, we will be able to reach our goal of providing excellent patient care in appropriate environments while providing the greatest flexibility and mobility with lightweight equipment. A comparison of the capabilities and personnel assets of combat hospitals is shown in Tables 16.2, 16.3, 16.4, and 16.5.

Major General Spurgeon Neel, one of the pioneers of helicopter air evacuation said, "Getting the casualties and the physician together is the keystone of the practice of combat medicine", but it is also the keystone of the practice of civilian medicine. In Vietnam and Korea, our mortality rates from battle casualties decreased significantly for a number of reasons. We were able to evacuate the patient rapidly to a well-equipped, well-staffed, and organized surgical hospital that was close to the combat zone. The composition of our hospi-

Table 16.2 Capabilities Comparison of Combat Hospitals

	MASH	CSH	EVAC
Beds (no.)	60	200	400
Operating rooms (no.)	4	4	6
Mobility (%)	100	35	25

Table 16.3 Comparison of Personnel Assets of Combat Hospitals

	MASH	CHS	EVAC
Total personnel	230	290	385
Officers (total)	66	71	87
Medical corps	16	18	24
Dental Corps	1	1	1
Nurse Corps	41	39	49
Medical Service Corps	6	9	9
Enlisted (total)	164	219	298
LVN	20	24	80
Aidmen	43	45	38
OR/CMS tech	25	27	32

Table 16.4 Comparison of Physician Assets of Combat Hospitals

Specialty	MASH	CHS	EVAC
General surgery	8	6	4
Thoracic surgery	1	1	1
Orthopedic surgery	3	2	4
Urology	—	—	—
OB-GYN	—	1	1
Anesthesiology	2	1	1
Ophthalmology	—	0	1
ENT	0	0	1
Neurosurgery	—	—	1
Emergency medicine	2	—	—
Internal medicine	—	3	3
General Medical Officer	—	2	3
Psychiatry	—	—	1
Radiology	—	1	1
Total	16	18	23

Table 16.5 Comparison of Nursing Assets of Combat Hospitals

	MASH	CHS	EVAC
Nurse administrator	1	1	1
Operating room nurse	9	6	7
Nurse anesthetist	7	4	6
Med-surg nurse	24	28	34
Psych/mental health nurse	0	0	1
Total	41	39	49

tals was tailored to fit the tactical situation. In the Second World War, air evacuation initially meant placing the patient in a small area of fixed-wing aircraft. During the Korean war, the helicopter became the mainstay of evacuation, but the patients were placed in pods on the outside of the aircraft and were totally isolated from any help. The UH-1H (Huey), which was used extensively in Vietnam, was originally designed to hold six litter patients but actually was able to hold only three litter patients and in some cases, because of climatic conditions, less.

The army has embarked on a plan to replace the Huey with a much improved helicopter. Sikorsky has designed the UH-60A, known as the Black Hawk. The helicopter in medical evacuation configuration has a crew of four and a single main rotor that is powered by two General Electric turbo shaft engines, each of which has 1,560 hp. It is 64.8 feet long, 17 feet high, can carry equipment either externally or internally, and, like all of our helicopters, the Black Hawk is almost double the weight of the Huey and has increased flexibility. It is more fuel efficient and a much safer aircraft. At 2,000 feet and 70 degrees Fahrenheit, the condition of a temperate climate, a Huey can lift three-quarters of a ton while a Black Hawk can lift 3 tons. Utilizing the Black Hawk, not only can we get a patient to a hospital more quickly but more patients can be transported. Six litter patients can be carried in a Huey, although three is the limit in a combat configuration, while four litter patients can be carried in a Black Hawk. Although initially this does not appear to be a major improvement, the major benefit that has been attained is total accessibility to the patient. There are 22 inches of free space for the top patient and in the lower litter rack there is 18 and one-half inches of free space. The Black Hawk also provides increased capacity for ambulatory patients over the Huey, depending on the mix of ambulatory and litter patients per load. The helicopter has a medical evacuation kit with oxygen, lights, and a power pack that will convert the current on the aircraft to 120 volts and 60 cycles and, therefore, permit a type of hospital equipment to be used in flight. Many new safety features have been built into the Black Hawk's design. It can sustain a 15-G crash, the superstructure has been strengthened, extra units have been added, and the fuel tanks and lines are self-sealing and have been located away from the underbelly as has wiring. The seats are load limiting, and there is an internal crash switch that activates a fire extinguishing system. The helicopter itself has increased maintainability; the Huey requires maintenance every 100 hours, the Black Hawk every 300 hours. The final results of these improvements are increased flexibility leading to a decrease in patient mortality and morbidity. From a medical standpoint, the major improvements are increase in payload capability, speed, range, and patient accessibility.

The U.S. Army has a continuing program of research and development to improve our medical capabilities. At Fort Sam Houston, Texas, the Academy of Health Sciences not only trains all of our medical personnel, be they physicians, nurses, or corpsmen, but in addition it has an organization that oversees and tests new equipment. Pure medical research is carried on by a number of units within the U.S. Army Medical Research and Development Command. The Uniformed Services University of the Health Sciences, a federal medical school housed on the campus of the Naval Regional Medical Center in Bethesda, Maryland, graduates approximately 150 medical students per year. They have a classical medical school curriculum, but in addition students are trained in the unique military aspects of medicine. During a medical student's four years at the university, they are exposed to all the uniformed services and have experience in not only fixed hospital facilities but in field units as well. The Division of Surgery at the University has ongoing research projects, in general and vascular trauma.

The University itself has a strong relationship with the research and development commands of the three services. The U.S. Army Medical Research and Development Command has three major facilities that deal in trauma. The first is the U.S. Army Institute of Surgical Research at Fort Sam Houston. Although this unit is usually known as the "burn unit", it is far more complex and carries on both research and treatment of trauma patients in general, in addition to burn research and treatment. Letterman Army Institute of Research is concentrating on blast injuries.

PART III
A STRATEGY FOR IMPLEMENTATION OF A REGIONAL TRAUMA SYSTEM

In the final section we will analyze some of the factors involved in establishing a regional trauma system. Chapter 17 attempts to analyze the impact of regionalization on trauma care. Our experience indicates that regions lacking an organized system of trauma care will have an unacceptable number of preventable deaths. It has yet to be demonstrated that implementation of a regional system of trauma care will decrease these deaths. We believe that the implementation of a regional trauma system will lead to a demonstrable decrease in the number of preventable deaths. This will provide strong support for the development of regional trauma systems in other parts of the country.

In Chapter 18 we will analyze two methods for evaluating regional trauma care. Our experience suggests that the key to the establishment of a regional trauma system is to convince the medical community that the current approach to trauma care results in an unacceptable number of preventable deaths. A simple, inexpensive, and remarkably accurate method is available to evaluate regional trauma care. This approach, which has been titled the "autopsy method," will be described in the first half of the chapter.

Despite the value of an autopsy study, our experience in Orange County was that a method relying solely on autopsy data did not have sufficient impact to convince the medical community to recommend a complete revision of our approach to trauma care. The study that was finally successful in convincing the Orange County medical community that trauma care must be restructured was based on a detailed analysis of both autopsy and hospital records. A method of performing such a clinical study will be outlined by Dr. Richard Cales in the remainder of the chapter.

No matter how well conceived a regional trauma plan may be, we can predict that there will be major barriers to its implementation. Dr. Charles R. McElroy examines the barriers faced with the implementation of a regional trauma plan for Los Angeles County in the following chapter. It is recognized that each region in this country will have its own unique problems, but Dr. McElroy has identified some of the major barriers that predictably will be found in almost every region.

The following chapter by John Fried, editor of the editorial section of the Long Beach Independent *Press/Telegram*, describes the role of an investigative reporter in evaluating the medical community's approach to trauma care. We felt it was important to include this chapter to demonstrate the role of the media in convincing the community that there is a need for an organized system of trauma care. The central point in establishing a regional trauma system is to have the regional trauma plan accepted by the local political body. Possibly more than anything else, the local political body will be responsive to public opinion. There is no better way to obtain favorable public opinion than by support from the news media. In this chapter, Mr. Fried clearly documents what a concerned investigative medical report can do to generate public support.

One of the first steps in establishing a regional trauma plan is to identify the major barriers to that plan. Once done, a strategy may be developed to overcome these barriers. In the closing statement we briefly outline the barriers to the establishment of the Orange County trauma plan and summarize the strategy used to overcome these barriers.

17
DO TRAUMA SYSTEMS SAVE LIVES?
John G. West, M.D.
Alan B. Gazzaniga, M.D.
Richard H. Cales, M.D.

It seems reasonable to assume that a region with an organized system of trauma care will do a better job of saving trauma victims than a region lacking such a system. Comparison between Orange County and San Francisco County in 1974 demonstrated that in Orange County, which lacked a system of trauma care, there was a high percentage of preventable deaths, whereas in San Francisco County, where there was an organized trauma care system, there were no preventable deaths.

To date we have, unfortunately, had little information regarding the quality of trauma care in a region before and after the designation of a regional trauma system. The question remains: To what extent does regionalization impact the quality of trauma care?

In an attempt to answer this question, we used the autopsy method to evaluate our first year's experience with a regional system of trauma care in Orange County.[1,2] We then compared this autopsy evaluation with two similar Orange County series that were evaluated prior to the designation of our regional trauma system. Our purpose was to evaluate the impact of regionalization on the quality of trauma care.

MATERIALS AND METHODS

In June, 1980, the Orange County trauma system was implemented. Five strategically located hospitals were designated as trauma centers. Each had agreed to provide an inhouse or immedi-

---

An adapted version of this chapter appeared in *Archives of Surgery* 118(6):740–44, 1983. Reprinted, with permission.

ately available trauma team around the clock. The university hospital was designated as the single Level I hospital according to the criteria of the American College of Surgeons[3] and inhouse coverage was provided by senior residents. Four community hospitals were designated as Level II. All patients were evaluated in the field by paramedics who obtained the vital signs and discussed their findings with the base station physician. Only those patients showing evidence of shock or cardiopulmonary distress were taken to the trauma center. It was the base station physician's responsibility to make this decision, and once made, the trauma center was notified that a patient was en route and the trauma team was mobilized.

Our review was limited to the deaths secondary to motor vehicular accidents for the period of June 15, 1980 to June 14, 1981. In accordance with the autopsy method, we eliminated prehospital deaths, DOAs (defined as field arrests with no vital signs on admission to the emergency room), and central nervous system deaths. We also eliminated four late deaths, since the original trauma was minimal and the cause of death was not related to the original injury (Table 17.1). In the remaining 29 deaths, the following information was obtained: (1) age of patient; (2) interval from injury to death; (3) whether the patient was taken to a trauma center, a nontrauma center, or transferred; (4) cause of death; and (5) whether an appropriate surgical procedure was performed. All deaths were independently reviewed by the three authors. Based on the above information, a decision was made as to whether or not the case was preventable. Unanimity was obtained on each death judged preventable.

The same method was applied to a similar group of traumatic deaths in Orange County (1974), Orange County (1978 to 1979), and San Francisco (1974). The results obtained in the present series were compared to the results obtained in the previous series. The purpose

Table 17.1 Four Late Deaths Eliminated from Series

1. Death secondary to pulmonary embolus longer than one month post multiple long bone fractures.

2. Death secondary to pulmonary embolus longer than two weeks post multiple long bone fractures.

3. Death secondary to fatty infiltration of liver; Injury was caused by a minor traffic collision.

4. Intrauterine death secondary to premature separation of placenta.

was to compare trauma survival with and without a system of trauma care.

Statistical analysis used the Fisher exact test. A p-value of less than 0.05 was required for statistical significance.

RESULTS

Three hundred and twenty motor vehicular-related trauma deaths occurred in Orange County during the period of study (Table 17.2). Although the total number of deaths and the number of central nervous system (CNS) deaths increased by 50 percent from the year 1974 to the years 1980 to 1981, the total number of non-CNS deaths occurring in Orange County during the first year following the implementation of a regional trauma system dropped slightly. During this first year, 944 patients met criteria and were sent to the trauma centers.

Twenty-nine fatally injured patients were included in the present study. Twenty-three patients were treated in a trauma center, four patients were treated in a nontrauma center, and two patients were transferred from a nontrauma center to a trauma center.

Survival

Two of twenty-three (9 percent) of the trauma center deaths were judged potentially preventable. These are summarized in Table 17.3. Two of the four deaths occurring in a nontrauma center were judged preventable and are summarized in Table 17.3. The remaining two deaths occurred in patients treated initially in a nontrauma center and subsequently transferred to a trauma center. Both deaths were judged preventable (Table 17.3).

Table 17.2   Orange County Trauma Deaths

	'74	'78-'79	'80-'81
CNS DEATHS	60	43*	96
NON-CNS DEATHS	30	21*	29
TOTAL TRAUMA DEATHS	218	317	320

*Represents stratified samples of CNS and NON-CNS deaths for yr. '78-'79.

Table 17.3   Preventable Deaths: Trauma Center vs Nontrauma Center

TRAUMA CENTER DEATHS			
AGE/SEX	INJURY	CAUSE OF DEATH	COMMENTS
22/male	Ruptured cecum	Sepsis	Unrecognized rupture of the cecum
70/male	Crushed chest, ruptured diaphragm	Pulmonary insufficiency	Missed rupture of diaphragm
NONTRAUMA CENTER DEATHS			
78/male	Lacerated portal vein	Hemorrhage	4 hrs. in ER - MI was suspected
66/male	Blunt trauma chest	Pulmonary insufficiency	Missed hemopneumothorax
TRANSFER FROM NONTRAUMA CENTER TO TRAUMA CENTER			
52/female	Lacerated liver, devascularized colon	Hemorrhage	Transferred to trauma center 36 hrs. post injury in profound shock
68/male	Liver laceration, avulsed gallbladder and pancreatitis	Hemorrhage, sepsis	3 days in nontrauma center; Sent to trauma center in profound shock

Of the 23 nonpreventable deaths, 10 died days to weeks following the original injury from complications of trauma such as sepsis, pulmonary insufficiency, or diffuse intravascular claudication (DIC). Seven additional deaths were secondary to major injuries involving the heart or thoracic aorta. Six of these seven cases had an operative attempt to control hemorrhage, although in most cases the operative procedure was an emergency room thoracotomy. The single exception was an 85-year-old male who had a cardiac arrest on arrival to the emergency room. In three cases the major injury was to the abdomen, and in each case there was an operative attempt to control hemorrhage. The remaining three deaths were secondary to crush injuries to the chest. In no case was there evidence of an unrecognized hemo- or pneumothorax or other apparently treatable condition.

In the previous two Orange County series (Table 17.4), 73 percent and 71 percent of the deaths were judged preventable and in the current series the percent of preventable deaths occurring in trauma centers was reduced to 9 percent. These differences are significant ($p < 0.001$). In patients sent initially to a nontrauma center, four out of six (67 percent) of the deaths were judged preventable. These differ-

Do Trauma Systems Save Lives?

Table 17.4 Comparison of Preventable Non-CNS Traumatic Deaths

Preventable Deaths

	S.F.-'74	O.C.-'74	O.C.-'78-'79	O.C.-'80-'81 Trauma Center	O.C.-'80-'81 Non Trauma Center
Preventable Deaths	0/16	22/30 73%	15/21 71%	2/23 9%	4/6 67%

▨ Represents regions with an organized system of trauma care.

ences in percentages of deaths occurring in a trauma center and nontrauma center are significant (p<0.01). Potentially preventable trauma center deaths in the current Orange County series (9 percent) approach the absence of preventable deaths noted in the 1974 San Francisco series. The 67 percent preventable deaths occurring in nontrauma centers are essentially the same in Orange County in the previous series, in which all patients were taken to the closest hospital rather than a trauma center.

Appropriate Surgery

We have suggested previously that in a trauma center setting, trauma victims requiring a life-saving operative procedure would be operated on.[4] In the present Orange County series, 23 patients required an immediate life-saving operative procedure. (Six other patients were eliminated. Five of these were patients with multiple fractures not requiring emergency surgery. The sixth was an elderly male whose aorta ruptured minutes after admission to the hospital.) Sixteen of eighteen (90 percent) of the patients taken to the trauma center received the appropriate operative procedure (Table 17.5). Only one of three patients taken to a nontrauma center received an appropriate operation. Of the two patients sent initially to a nontrauma center and later transferred to a trauma center, one was operated on and the other was not. In the case operated on, a devascularized right colon was missed and the hemorrhage was not controlled. We concluded that the appropriate operation was not performed. Therefore, only one of five (20 percent) of the patients taken to a nontrauma center received an appropriate surgical procedure. These differences between the percentage of appropriate operations performed in a trauma center and a nontrauma center are significant (p<0.01).

Table 17.5 Comparison of Non-CNS Traumatic Deaths Where Appropriate Surgery Was Performed

Appropriate Surgery

	S.F.-'74	O.C.-'74	O.C.-'78-'79	O.C.-'80-'81 Trauma Center	O.C.-'80-'81 Non Trauma Center
Appropriate Operation Performed	15/16 94%	6/30 20%	3/21 14%	16/18 89%	1/5 20%

▨ Represents regions with an organized system of trauma care.

In the previous two Orange County series, 20 percent and 14 percent of the patients received an appropriate surgical procedure, whereas in the current series, 89 percent of the patients taken to a trauma center received the appropriate surgical procedure. These differences are significant ($p < 0.001$). Further comparison of the present Orange County series with the previous series yields some striking parallels. In the current series, 89 percent of the patients taken to a trauma center received the appropriate surgical procedure. This is remarkably similar to the 94 percent noted in the 1974 San Francisco series. In the current series, when patients were taken to the nontrauma centers, only 20 percent received the appropriate surgical procedure. This is close to the 20 percent and 14 percent noted in the previous Orange County series before the designation of trauma centers.

Hemorrhage

We would expect that patients hemorrhaging on arrival to the trauma center would be operated on. In the present series, this was the case in 14 of 16 patients presenting with life-threatening hemorrhage (Table 17.6). Only one of these fourteen patients seen at the trauma centers did not have the appropriate operation. This was an 85-year-old male who arrested shortly after admission with a ruptured thoracic aorta. One of the two patients with life-threatening hemorrhage received the appropriate surgical procedure in a nontrauma center. These differences between percent of patients operated on to control hemorrhage in a trauma center and a nontrauma center are not statistically significant.

In the two previous Orange County series, 57 percent and 67 percent of the patients who died secondary to hemorrhage did not have an appropriate surgical procedure to control hemorrhage. In the

Table 17.6 Comparison of Non-CNS Traumatic Deaths from Hemorrhage

Hemorrhage and Surgery

	S.F.-'74	O.C.-'74	O.C.-'78-'79	O.C.-'80-'81 Trauma Center	O.C.-'80-'81 Non Trauma Center
Hemorrhagic Deaths (no surgery performed)	1/16 6%	17/30 57%	14/21 67%	1/14 7%	1/2 50%

▨ Represents regions with an organized system of trauma care.

present series, 7 percent of the patients who suffered a hemorrhagic death did not have a surgical procedure in an attempt to control the hemorrhage. These differences are significant ($p < 0.005$).

Again, we note some rather striking parallels when we compare the present Orange County series with the previous series. The percentage of hemorrhagic deaths without surgical intervention occurring in a trauma center is essentially the same in the present Orange County series as it was in the San Francisco series. Although the numbers are quite small, the percentage of hemorrhagic deaths without appropriate surgical intervention in the nontrauma centers in the present series was approximately the same as it was in the two previous series prior to the designation of the trauma system. The number of hemorrhagic deaths occurring in each series is depicted in Figure 17.1. It is clear that in the two series lacking an organized system of trauma care (Orange County 1974; Orange County 1978 to 1979) the majority of deaths were related to hemorrhage and that in the cases dying a hemorrhagic death the majority did not have an appropriate surgical procedure in an attempt to control the hemorrhage.

Age and Interval from Injury to Death

In a previous publication,[2] we suggested that in a trauma center setting, after excluding deaths from injuries to the heart or great vessels, the majority of trauma victims alive on arrival to the trauma center would live more than six hours. We found no statistically significant changes in this variable following the institution of the trauma system in Orange County. We also suggested that in the trauma center setting, death in patients under 50 years of age would be less common, and, therefore, one would expect a higher percent-

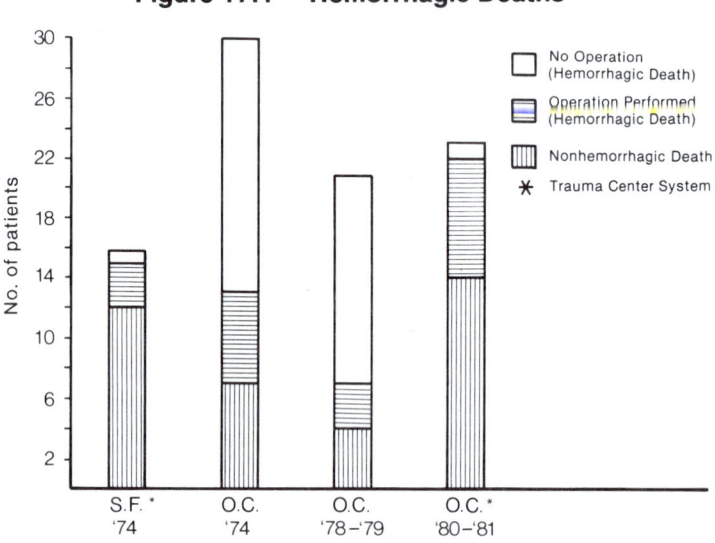

Figure 17.1 Hemorrhagic Deaths

Comparison between care at a trauma center and a non trauma center with respect to a) surgery performed to control hemorrhaging. b) proportion of hemorrhagic and non hemorrhagic deaths.

age of deaths in patients over 50 years of age. Following designation of trauma centers in Orange County, we found no significant change in the proportion of patients dying over 50 years of age (Table 17.7).

Discussion

Survival

Combining the results of all the studies, past and present, described in this chapter, we note of 39 patients delivered to a trauma center, two (5 percent) died a potentially preventable death. On the other hand, of 57 patients delivered to a nontrauma center, 41 (72 percent) died needlessly. The results suggest that trauma centers encourage aggressive surgical management and survival of critically injured trauma victims.

Autopsy Method

Our experience illustrates several advantages of the autopsy method of trauma care assessment. The first is simplicity. A survey

Table 17.7 Comparison of Non-CNS Traumatic Deaths with Arrival Time and Age as a Factor in Survival

Arrival Time and Age as a Factor in Survival

	S.F.-'74	O.C.-'74	O.C.-'78-'79	O.C.-'80-'81
Death less than six hours of arrival to ER (exclude injuries to heart and great vessels)	4/16 25%	21/30 70%	14/21 67%	8/20 40%
Death in patients older than 50 years	12/16 75%	6/30 20%	8/21 38%	12/29 41%

▨ Represents regions with an organized system of trauma care.

can be easily performed in fewer than 50 man-hours per two million total population. Second, it requires little money since it makes use primarily of public records. Third, although the method deals with a complex problem, it extracts a few prime indicators that can be relatively easily evaluated, such as cause of death and whether or not the appropriate operation was performed. These appear to be the key factors in evaluating any trauma system.

Thus, the autopsy method provides a means by which communities can evaluate trauma care in their regions. If, for example, a community were to find a majority of cases had an appropriate operation, deaths were occurring days to weeks following admission from complications of trauma, primarily in elderly individuals, they would have strong evidence to suggest adequate trauma care.

There are distinct limitations to the autopsy method. It cannot be used to evaluate prehospital care, since prehospital deaths are eliminated. It is of limited value in evaluating resuscitative efforts, since the timing of the resuscitative efforts and the volume of fluid and blood replaced cannot be determined. There is no way to evaluate the time of arrival of the appropriate consultant. A further limitation is that it is impossible to evaluate the timing of surgical intervention. The latter issue is of particular concern, since the method essentially assumes that if surgery is performed, it is done on a timely basis. The situations in which delay of surgery contributes to the death are not recognized by the method. Intraoperative judgment and operative skills cannot be accurately assessed. Postoperative care can be only very superficially evaluated. Since most patients who die days to weeks following injury are judged to be nonpreventable, the method tends to underestimate the number of potentially preventable deaths.[4] In spite of these limitations, the autopsy method serves its goal—to uncover major deficiencies in trauma care in a given community.

Problems of Triage

A major area of concern highlighted by this study was the fact that 21 percent ($6/29$) of trauma victims were sent to a nontrauma center. Two-thirds of such deaths were judged potentially preventable, whereas only 9 percent of the patients sent to a trauma center were so judged. These findings underscore the necessity of identifying in the field those patients whose proper destination is a trauma center. In patients in shock with obvious hypotension, the problem is straightforward.

Unfortunately, many patients with serious intraabdominal or intrathoracic injuries may look deceptively stable when first seen by the paramedics. The correct identification of patients with major injuries who are seen before they reflect the earliest hemodynamic responses of shock will be impossible if one relies solely on the vital signs.

Some authors have attempted to define quantitatively the decision regarding triage by scoring physiological and clinical parameters in a semiquantitative fashion.[5,6] In Orange County, we adopted a more qualitative triage protocol. Any patient with evidence of shock or cardiopulmonary distress is a candidate for triage to the trauma center. Our current experience suggests that methods that rely primarily on vital signs and clinical assessment will result in approximately 20 percent of the patients with serious injuries being incorrectly sent to a nontrauma center.

To identify the group with serious injuries in spite of stable vital signs requires consideration of mechanism of injury. In other words, one must evaluate not only the patient but the accident itself to determine if the forces involved were of sufficient magnitude to cause serious injury. Such examples might include high-speed motor vehicle accidents. In accidents in which one victim was killed outright, the other victim should be sent to the trauma center. If a person was ejected from an auto, he or she should be considered at high risk for serious injury. Finally, any patient over 60 years of age should be considered for triage to a trauma center in any but the most trivial of automobile accidents.

In situations where the mechanism of injury is judged to be of major magnitude, victims should be taken to a trauma center despite stable vital signs. If the magnitude of injury is judged to be intermediate, triage to the trauma center should be based on evaluation of the patient. When the patient is seen within the first few minutes of injury, it is essential to look for the earliest signs of shock, such as pallor, diaphoresis, and subtle abnormalities of the pulse or respiratory rate. If the mechanism of injury is of intermediate severity and the victim shows even the most subtle signs of shock, he or she should be transferred to a trauma center. No matter what the criteria, some degree of overtriage (defined as a hospital stay of less than three days) is inevitable. Similarly, undertriage (in which victims of major trauma will be sent to a nontrauma center) will occur. With an effective trauma system, the percentage of overtriage cases should be less than 30 percent of the total number of cases sent to the trauma center. Undertriage, i.e., the percent of trauma deaths occurring in nontrauma centers, should be less than 5 percent of all trauma deaths.

SUMMARY

This chapter demonstrates a significant reduction in the number of preventable deaths following the implementation of a regional trauma system. Additionally, it demonstrated a more aggressive approach to trauma victims in terms of performing the appropriate surgical procedure.

We feel that these data should have widespread applicability. Regions lacking an organized system of trauma care can anticipate an unacceptable number of preventable deaths. Organization of the community's resources, such as the triage of critical trauma victims to a designated trauma center and evaluation by skilled physicians on a timely basis, will markedly limit the number of preventable deaths. Communities that have yet to organize trauma care systems can ill afford to ignore this message. This tragic loss of young lives can be avoided by a logical utilization of available community resources.

ACKNOWLEDGEMENT

We wish to thank Dr. Leonard Berman, who reviewed this manuscript and provided many valuable suggestions and criticisms.

REFERENCES

1. West, JG: An autopsy method for evaluation trauma care. *J. Trauma* 21:32, 1981.
2. West, JG: A validation of the autopsy method. *Arch. Surg.* 117:1033, 1982.
3. Optimum Hospital Resources for the Care of the Injured Patient. Bulletin, American College of Surgeons, August, 1979.
4. West, JG, Trunkey, DD, Lim, RC: Systems of trauma care: A study of two counties. *Arch. Surg.* 114:445, 1979.
5. Champion, HR, Sacco, WJ, Carnazzo, AJ: The trauma score. *Crit. Care Med.* 9:672, 1981.
6. Gormican, SP: Crams scale—Field triage of trauma victims. *Ann. Emerg. Med.* 2:132, 1982.

18
METHODS OF EVALUATION OF TRAUMA CARE
John G. West, M.D.
Richard H. Cales, M.D.

Our experience in Orange County has led us to the conclusion that the key to establishing a regional trauma system is the demonstration that in regions lacking such a system, young healthy trauma victims are dying needlessly. In this chapter we will describe two separate methods of analyzing regional trauma care: the autopsy and the clinical methods. The first will be the autopsy method, which is simple and inexpensive since it is based on the autopsy and coroner's report, both of which are a matter of public record.[1]

THE AUTOPSY METHOD

The first step in the process of data collection is to obtain records for the most recently available series of motor vehicle deaths using ICDA codes E-810 through E-819 (Table 18.1). Five hundred consecutive deaths are optimal, although in sparsely populated areas a smaller sample is acceptable. Patients who are obviously dead on arrival are eliminated from this series. Central nervous system (CNS) deaths should also be eliminated, since salvageability is more difficult to determine in these cases without hospital records. Autopsy records and coroner's reports are then obtained for the remaining 50 to 100 cases.

This data base provides the (1) age, (2) time interval from arrival at the hospital to death, (3) whether or not an operation was performed, and (4) the cause of death.

Table 18.1 The Autopsy Method: Data Base

1. Evaluate 500 consecutive death certificates from victims of motor vehicular trauma ICD-9-CM Codes E-810 through E-819.
2. Eliminate prehospital deaths, DOAs, and CNS deaths.
3. Autopsy reports, coroners' reports, and death certificates of the remaining 50 to 100 cases provide the following data:
   age of patient
   time from arrival at hospital until death
   laparotomy or thoracotomy performed
   cause of death

Certain key points may then be evaluated (Table 18.2). It has been noted by Baker and colleagues that for a given magnitude of injury, mortality is noticeably higher for patients aged 50 to 69 years and increases sharply in patients over 70.[2,3] One should, therefore, pay particular attention to deaths occurring in patients less than 50 years of age, since they are more easily salvaged. Attention should also be focused on patients dying less than six hours after arrival in the emergency room (excluding those patients who died secondary to injury of the heart and/or great vessels). Finally, all deaths secondary to exsanguination should be carefully evaluated, with particular emphasis on those patients who did not undergo an operative procedure to control hemorrhage.

These warning signs taken in context may serve to identify preventable deaths. For example, a young trauma victim who exsanguinates from a ruptured spleen two hours after arrival in the emergency room and who is not operated on would be considered a preventable death. If in the same example the exsanguination was from a ruptured thoracic aorta, the death would almost certainly not be judged preventable. The warning signs serve to identify those deaths that are at high risk of being preventable. The final judgment as to whether or not a death is preventable should not be made until all available clinical data have been carefully evaluated.

Using the above method, we have published a comparison study of Orange County, where there was no system of trauma care, and San Francisco County, with its highly structured system of trauma care.[4] We reviewed 30 non-CNS deaths from Orange County and 16 non-CNS deaths from San Francisco during a similar time period. The majority of trauma deaths in the Orange County series occurred in patients less than 50 years of age, whereas the majority of deaths in the San Francisco series were in patients over 50 years of age (Figure 18.1).

Table 18.2 The Autopsy Method: Warning Signs

1. Deaths in patients less than 50 years of age
2. Time interval from arrival at hospital to time of death, less than 6 hours, excluding cases with injury to the heart or great vessels
3. Failure to perform laparotomy or thoracotomy
4. Hemorrhagic deaths

The time interval from arrival at the hospital to the time of death also showed a distinct difference between the two series. In Orange County, 24 of 30 patients died within six hours of arrival at the emergency room (3 of the patients probably should have been excluded because of injuries to the heart and/or great vessels). In contrast, the majority of deaths in the San Francisco series occurred several days after admission.

The cause of death was also markedly different in the two series. In Orange County 23 of 30 deaths were from hemorrhagic shock, while in San Francisco only 4 such deaths occurred. The remaining 12 deaths in the San Francisco series were attributed to progressive pulmonary insufficiency or multisystem organ failure. In Orange County, only 6 of 30 patients were operated on, whereas in San Francisco, 15 of 16 patients received an appropriate operative procedure. Utilizing the above data, 22 of 30 deaths in the Orange County series were judged preventable; in San Francisco, no preventable deaths were found (Table 18.3).

We attempted to assess the accuracy of the autopsy method in a follow-up study. In 1979, the Orange County Board of Supervisors and the Orange County Medical Association sponsored a study of 100 inhospital motor vehicle deaths using clinical and autopsy records. Results indicated that 18 or 21 (85 percent) of the non-CNS patients studied were potentially salvageable.[5] We independently evaluated these 21 non-CNS patients using the autopsy method and concluded that 16 of 21 (72 percent) were preventable.[6] Each death judged preventable by the autopsy method was also judged preventable by the more detailed hospital records method. Therefore, no false positives were noted by the autopsy method.

The hospital records method did judge 3 deaths preventable that were judged not preventable by the autopsy method. The first was a 17-year-old boy with a transected thoracic aorta who was stable for 36 hours before dying of hemorrhagic shock. The second patient was a 51-year-old man with liver and lung lacerations who died 18 minutes after arrival at the emergency room. Volume replacement was

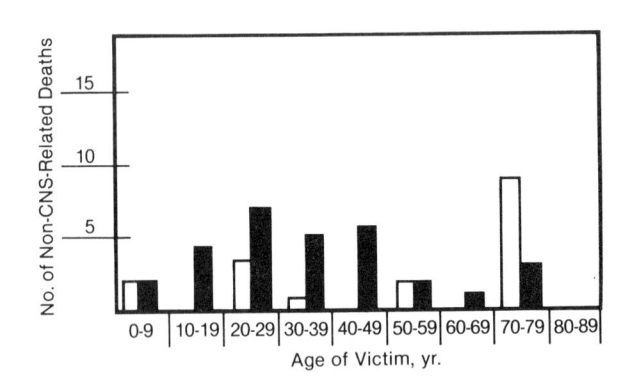

Figure 18.1 The Autopsy Method: Age Distributions.

Age distributions for Orange County series deaths (solid bars) and San Francisco County series deaths (open bars). (Reprinted with permission from West, J. G., Trunkey, D. D., Lim, R. C.: Systems of trauma care: A study of two counties. *Arch. Surg.*, **114:** 445–460, 1979).

totally inadequate. The final patient was a 61-year-old man with pelvic fractures and a lacerated superficial femoral artery. There were delays in control of bleeding resulting in extensive blood loss and eventual death from disseminated intravascular coagulation and renal failure.

It is not surprising that the autopsy method is at risk for false negatives, since pertinent clinical materials regarding resuscitative efforts, timing of surgery, and judgment are not available for review. We conclude that the autopsy method is an effective screening method for evaluation of trauma care, but that it understates the problem it exposes.

THE CLINICAL METHOD

A second approach to the evaluation of regional trauma care is the clinical method, which, although more expensive and time consuming, is also more precise because it additionally utilizes the prehospital and hospital records.

The clinical method of evaluation of the quality of trauma care follows a logical sequence, including definition of the patient population, identification of the physician reviewers, assembly of the necessary data, documentation of system and medical care, quantification of the degree of injury, and calculation of death rates. Based on this

Table 18.3 The Autopsy Method: Potentially Preventable Deaths

Patient/Sex/Age (years)	Trauma	Cause of Death	Comment
1/M/51	Ruptured spleen; lacerated mesenteric artery	Hemorrhage	Patient observed 2 hours
2/F/25	Ruptured spleen	Hemorrhage	Interhospital transfer delayed definitive care; patient died 1 hour 45 minutes after injury
3/M/30	Lacerated liver	Hemorrhage	Patient died 1 hour 45 minutes after injury
4/M/5	Lacerated liver	Hemorrhage	Presumed diagnosis of CNS-related injury not confirmed on postmortem examination; patient died 1 hour 15 minutes after arrival in emergency room
5/M/75	Ruptured spleen; lacerated lung; tibial-fibular fracture	Hemorrhage	Cardiac arrest 2 hours after injury while fracture being set
6/M/51	Lacerated spleen; multiple long bone fractures	Hemorrhage	Patient observed in emergency room for 1 hour 45 minutes
7/F/76	Perforated small bowel	Sepsis	Patient observed in hospital for 36 hours
8/M/48	Lacerated mesenteric artery	Hemorrhage	Presumed diagnosis of ruptured aorta; thoracotomy performed
9/F/24	Blunt trauma to chest	Pericardial tamponade	Cardiac arrest in intensive care unit 3 days after injury; postmortem examination revealed 400 ml liquid blood in pericardial sac; hemorrhage predated cardiac arrest
10/M/41	Lacerated liver	Hemorrhage	Patient observed in emergency room for 45 minutes; no resuscitation attempted; patient died 1 hour 10 minutes after injury
11/M/20	Lacerated liver	Exsanguination	Liver laceration closed with surface sutures; massive intrahepatic hematoma developed; patient died 5 hours 25 minutes after admission

Source: Reprinted with permission from West, J.G., Trunkey, D.D., Lim, R.C.: Systems of trauma care: A study of two counties. *Arch. Surg.*, 114: 445–460, 1979.

information the reviewers then assess the appropriateness of outcome (Table 18.4).

One of the advantages of the clinical method is the opportunity it provides for broad-based participation by physicians, hospitals, and prehospital personnel. Experience has shown that such joint sponsorship by the medical association, hospital council, and emergency medical services (EMS) system is instrumental in establishing the credibility of the evaluation process and the resulting recommendations for the modification of trauma care.

The first step in the process of data collection, which is identical to that of the autopsy method, is to obtain records for the most recently available series of motor vehicle deaths using ICD-9-CM codes E-810 through E-819. Two hundred and fifty to three hundred consecutive cases are optimal, as this should provide one hundred cases after the appropriate exlusions. (Fewer cases are required by the clinical method, because it does not exlude CNS deaths.)

The first screening phase consists of review of police and coroner's records to exclude those patients who could not be reasonably expected to benefit from improvements in trauma care (prehospital cardiac arrests, patients injured in other counties, and patients dying of burns not associated with blunt or penetrating trauma). Following this process, a random selection may be desirable to reduce the study sample to a more practical number. In the second screening phase, the prehospital and hospital record is additionally reviewed, again excluding those patients who fail to meet the original criteria.

The clinical audit, including the prehospital and hospital chart evaluation, is performed by teams of physician specialists, consisting of general surgeons, neurosurgeons, and emergency physicians. Appointment of these individuals by their respective specialty societies is desirable in order to remove any potential selection bias.

Each physician reviewer is supplied with a comprehensive data base, including coroner's records, prehospital records, and the hospital chart (Table 18.5). Access to the hospital chart may be achieved by conferring temporary staff privileges on physician reviewers who may then examine the clinical record in the medical records depart-

Table 18.4   The Clinical Method: Steps in Evaluation

1. Patient selection
2. Physician reviewer selection
3. Medical and system audit
4. Determination of injury severity score
5. Determination of death rates
6. Physician assessment of appropriateness of outcome

Table 18.5 The Clinical Method: Data Base

Paramedic field record	Coroner's investigation
Paramedic base station record	Coroner's autopsy
Hospital chart	Death certificate

ment of the hospital(s) where the patients were treated. This method avoids the necessity of reproducing hospital charts and provides an additional layer of legal protection from discovery of confidential medical information.

The evaluation of system and medical care is conducted according to objective criteria supplied to each physician reviewer in the form of a multi-page worksheet, which is summarized in Table 18.6. Epidemiologic data include the age and sex of the victim and the etiology and location of the incident. Time intervals in the field and hos-

Table 18.6 The Clinical Method: Audit Criteria by Category.

Epidemiologic Data
  Hospital(s) coded
  Patient (coded)
  Age/sex/race
  Date of injury
  Date of death
  Etiology of injury
  Location of injury
  Cause of death
Time Factors
  Injury
  Arrival of advanced life support (ALS)
  Transport
  Admission to emergency department
  Blood administration
  Consultant arrival
  Emergency department surgical intervention
  Operating room surgical intervention
  Cardiac arrest
  Death
Treatment
  Prehospital
    Resuscitation ABCs
    Musculoskeletal stabilization
    Neurologic evaluation
    Fluid resuscitation
  Emergency
    Monitoring
    Fluid resuscitation
    Diagnostic intervention
    Consultant availability
    Therapeutic intervention
  Operative
    Hemostasis
    Fluid resuscitation
    Monitoring
    Procedures
  Postop
    Monitoring
    Rehabilitation

pital are documented to evaluate the effect of delays in prehospital resuscitation, transport, and diagnosis and treatment. The clinical evaluation of each case includes identification of diagnostic and therapeutic procedures in the prehospital, emergency department, operative, and postoperative phases of care.

The prehospital phase requires evaluation of response times of paramedical personnel, appropriate evaluation and application of basic life support techniques followed by musculoskeletal stabilization, judicious use of fluid resuscitation and the pneumatic antishock garment, and timely evacuation to the nearest qualified medical facility. Once in the emergency department, attention is focused upon continuing advanced life support, resuscitation with intravenous fluids and blood, and institution of appropriate diagnostic and therapeutic procedures, such as tube thoracostomy, peritoneal lavage, and pericardiocentesis. Special attention must be given to documentation of prompt availability of general and specialty surgical consultation and immediate access to properly staffed and equipped surgical suites. Evaluation of the operative phase includes continuing volume resuscitation with fluids and blood and institution of appropriate surgical procedures. Postoperative assessment examines continuing blood loss and monitoring and management of medical complications.

Quantitative assessment of the degree of injury may be determined by a severity scoring system, such as that of the American College of Surgeons in its Hospital Trauma Index[7] or the American Association for Automotive Medicine in AIS-80.[8] Based on this comprehensive body of objective information, each physician reviewer provides a subjective evaluation as to the appropriateness of outcome in each case. This evaluation of "potential salvageability" is made by comparing actual care rendered to that of an "optimal trauma system" with immediately available surgery and anesthesia. Although such a capability may not have existed at the time of treatment, the definition provides a uniform standard of comparison for the purpose of evaluation. In addition to the clinical chart review, the study should include an evaluation of mortality rates obtained from the state.

Numerous clinical studies have previously used similar methods to evaluate the appropriateness of outcome and the potential for improvement under a different system of care.[9-26] Each of these reports, however, has addressed a single time interval, and none has studied a comparable patient population following implementation of the proposed improvements.

Methods of Evaluation

In 1982, we used the clinical method to evaluate the mortality of trauma before and after the June, 1980, implementation of a comprehensive trauma system in Orange County.[27] The patient selection was accomplished in two phases as described above (Table 18.7), resulting in 58 and 60 cases, respectively, for each of the pre- and postsystem audits. At the conclusion of the study we found statistically significant improvements in trauma care in every area subjected to examination (Table 18.8). Following implementation of the system the proportion of potentially salvageable deaths dropped from 34 percent to 15 percent, with the overwhelming majority of the potentially salvageable deaths (78 percent) occurring in a minority of patients (22 percent) who were not sent to trauma facilities.

The median age of patients dying of trauma rose from 22 to 27 years of age while the median injury severity score rose from 42 to 52. In addition, the Orange County death rate fell from a projected value of 15.72 deaths per 100,000 population to 13.93 deaths per 100,000, while no other surrounding area showed a comparable drop in trauma mortality.

We conclude that the clinical method has demonstrated that implementation of a trauma system has had a significant impact on the

Table 18.7 The Clinical Method: Patient Selection

	1977–1978	1980–1981
Total motor vehicular accident deaths	317	320
Excluded (coroner, police records)*	134	153
Patients subjected to randomization	183	167
Random sample	100	100
Excluded (hospital records)*	42	40
Included in final report	58	60

*Exclusions: prehospital cardiac arrests, out-of-county injuries, burns not associated with trauma

Table 18.8 The Clinical Method: Results

	1977–1978	1980–1981	Significant
Proportion of potentially salvageable patients dying of trauma	34%	15%	$p < 0.02$
Median age of patients dying of trauma	22	27	$p < 0.05$
Median ISS of patients dying of trauma	42	52	$p < 0.025$
System error (multiple categories)	(poor)	(good)	—
Deaths/100,000 population from vehicular trauma	15.72	13.93	$p < 0.03$

quality of trauma care in Orange County. Emphasis must now be placed on further reduction in system error through refinement of triage criteria, which will minimize the incidence of trauma death outside trauma facilities. Issues of morbidity, cost, and the relative contribution of individual components within the system remain to be addressed by a prospective study.

SUMMARY

Trauma care requires the development of highly specialized systems that must be developed and implemented on a local basis based on demonstrated need and available resources. The autopsy and clinical methods of evaluation of trauma have been described as they relate to the development and medical audit of trauma systems.

REFERENCES

1. West, JG: An autopsy method for evaluating trauma care. *J. Trauma* 21:32, 1981.
2. Baker, SP, O'Neill, B: The injury severity score: A method for describing patients with multiple injuries and evaluating emergency care. *J. Trauma* 14:187, 1974.
3. Baker, SP, O'Neill, B: The injury severity score: An update. *J. Trauma* 16:882, 1976.
4. West, JG, Trunkey, DD, Lim, RC: Systems of trauma care: A study of two counties. *Arch. Surg.* 114:455, 1979.
5. Report to the Orange County Board of Supervisors: 1979 Trauma System Care Study.
6. West, JG: Validation of autopsy method for evaluating trauma care. *Arch. Surg.* 117:1033, 1982.
7. Hospital Resources for Optimal Care of the Seriously Injured. Trauma Appendices. Bulletin, American College of Surgeons, February, 1980, pp. 31–33.
8. Abbreviated Injury Scale (rev.) American Association for Automotive Medicine, Morton Grove, Illinois, 1980.
9. Detmer, DE, Moylan, JA, Rose, J, Schulz, R, Wallace, R, Daly, R: Regional categorization and quality of care in major trauma. *J. Trauma* 17:592, 1977.
10. Dove, DB, Stahl, WM, del Guercio, LRM: A five-year review of deaths following urban trauma. *J. Trauma* 20:760, 1980.
11. Foley, RW, Harris, LS, Pilcher, DB: Abdominal injuries in automobile accidents: Review of fatally injured patients. *J. Trauma* 17:611, 1977.
12. Fitts, WT, Lehr, HB, Bitner, RL, Spelman, JW: An analysis of 950 fatal injuries. *Surgery* 56:663, 1964.
13. Frey, CF, Huelke, DF, Gikas, PW: Resuscitation and survival in motor vehicle accidents. *J. Trauma* 9:292, 1969.
14. Gertner, HR, Baker, SP, Rutherford, RB, Spitz, WU: Evaluation of the management of vehicular fatalities secondary to abdominal injury. *J. Trauma* 12:425, 1972.

15. Gill, W, Champion, HR, Long, WB, Stega, M, Nolan, J, Decker, R, Misinscky, M, Cowley, RA: A clinical experience of major multiple trauma in Maryland. *Maryland State Med. J.* 25:55, 1976.

16. Gilmore, KM, Clemmer, TP, Orme, JF: Commitment to trauma in a low population density area. *J. Trauma* 21:883, 1981.

17. Houtchens, BA: Major trauma in the rural mountain West. *J.A.C.E.P.* 6:343, 1977.

18. Moylan, JA, Detmer, DE, Rose, J, Schulz, R: Evaluation of the quality of hospital care in major trauma. *J. Trauma* 16:517, 1976.

19. Perry, JF, McClellan, RJ: Autopsy findings in 127 patients following fatal traffic accidents. *Surg. Gyn. Obstet.* 119:586, 1964.

20. Root, GT, Christensen, BH: Early surgical treatment of abdominal injuries in the traffic victim. *Surg. Gyn. Obstet.* 105:264, 1957.

21. Trunkey, DD, Lim, RC: Analysis of 425 consecutive trauma facilities: An autopsy study. *J.A.C.E.P.* 3:368, 1974.

22. Van Wagoner, FH: Died in hospital: A three-year study of deaths following trauma. *J. Trauma* 1:401, 1961.

23. Waller, JA, Curran, R, Noyes, F: Traffic deaths: A preliminary study of urban and rural fatalities in California. *Cal. Med.* 101:272, 1964.

24. Waller, JA: Urban-oriented methods: Failure to solve rural emergency care problems. *J.A.M.A.* 226:1441, 1973.

25. Waters, JM, Wells, CH: The effects of a modern emergency medical service system in reducing automobile crash deaths. *J. Trauma* 13:645, 1973.

26. Zollinger, RW: Traffic injuries: A surgical problem. *Arch. Surg.* 70:694, 1955.

27. Cales, RH: Trauma mortality: The effect of implementation of a regional trauma system (submitted to *New Eng. J. Med.*), 1982.

19
OBSTRUCTIONS IN THE ROAD TO TRAUMA CARE: THE LOS ANGELES EXPERIENCE
Charles R. McElroy, M.D.

RECOGNITION OF A PROBLEM IN THE
CARE OF TRAUMA VICTIMS

Accidental death is the leading cause of death in the United States of America for citizens up to the thirty-seventh year. One hundred fifteen thousand persons were fatally injured in 1971; 54,764 of these deaths related specifically to motor vehicle accidents. In terms of statistics, one out of four Americans was injured at work or play during 1971 and the overall cost of these accidents to the nation was approximately thirty billion dollars. Of the 52 million citizens injured annually, 11 million required bed care for a day or more, and 40,000 suffered long-term disability. Those patients hospitalized occupy approximately 65,000 beds for 22 million bed-days under the care of 88,000 hospital personnel; a load which is equivalent to 3,500 bed hospitals.[1]

Although the statistical and economic magnitude of the problem is well recognized, little has been done to improve deficiencies in trauma care.

The facilities and knowledge to halve the mortality rate are available, but require drastic reorganization. Much attention has been directed at educating the public, improving first aid at the scene of injury and during transport to the hospital. To date, the care offered by the receiving physician has avoided scrutiny, yet this aspect of emergency health care delivery is frequently deficient. Be it as a result of poor planning by senior physicians or lack of training by junior staff, many lives are lost as a result of inadequate medical care.[1]

In support of these allegations, a number of studies have shown that many victims of trauma die as a result of inadequate medical systems or inadequate individual medical care.

> A Vermont study found that approximately half of the motor vehicle related deaths occurring in hospitals resulted from injuries potentially salvageable. In Philadelphia, 51 injury deaths involved errors in diagnosis or management. In Baltimore, it was found that 50 percent of patients who succumbed to abdominal injuries might have survived with better management, closer observation, and better communication. A third of the deaths involved grossly inadequate management of hypovolemic shock. In today's demanding society it is apparent that physicians must improve their ability to cope with life-threatening injury by attending to the basic principles which are so frequently ignored in practice.[1]

In our own area, Drs. Trunkey and West deflated both the public confidence and the medical ego by publishing data that reflected on trauma care in Orange and San Francisco Counties in the 1970s. This study showed that the majority of patients treated at that time in Orange County who died as a result of trauma could have been saved. On release of the information, both public and medical outcry was vigorous and denial rather universal. To prove that the data were unsound, a repeat study was done and, to my knowledge, never reported. However, shortly thereafter, a trauma system was evolved and put in place in Orange County.

Stimulated by the Trunkey-West study, the UCLA Emergency Medicine group led by Dr. Orban, using the Trunkey-West model, studied 100 trauma deaths in Los Angeles County. Not surprisingly, the reviewers again concluded that the majority of trauma deaths in Los Angeles County were also preventable. It is important to emphasize that most of the victims in these studies died of relatively straightforward problems such as hypovolemic shock, ruptured spleens, and a variety of other injuries that would be easily managed by any experienced trauma team.

I strongly suggest that review of trauma care leads to the inevitable conclusion that considerable improvements can and should be made. However, it is a sad but valid fact that perhaps the least-organized and least-progressive group in developing training programs in accident surgery are the physicians themselves. Although scattered centers throughout both the United States and other countries exist, where high-quality trauma programs occur, the vast majority of the medical profession do not appear fully aware of the magnitude of the problem.

> How curious that this problem of trauma which by actuarial analysis is the leading cause of death and disability of all age groups is almost totally absent from the medical student curriculum and appears only sporadically, and somewhat half-heartedly, in most resident and registrar surgical training programs. How curious that one of the three most important killers of man is not regarded as sufficiently important to be granted the formal status of a distinct medical specialty. Progress in the medical reception, resuscitation, and management of the seriously injured will continue to be slow and faltering until these anachronisms are rectified.[1]

One might ask why there has been no recognition or why recognition of the problem has been actively repressed. There are many reasons, and I will mention several. First of all, many medical personnel, hospital administrators, and other involved individuals genuinely feel that they and the system are doing a good job. Lack of effective review, lack of access to records of trauma victims, lack of effective charting during resuscitation of seriously injured individuals as well as fear of litigation and lack of expectation of a good outcome for trauma victims all come together to produce the apathy that abounds in the medical community.

All of us would certainly investigate the death of a middle-aged successful executive scheduled for elective surgery who used a hospital of choice, a surgeon of excellent reputation, and succumbed as a result of some untoward event during the surgery. No one under these circumstances simply accepts the death as an unfortunate occurrence. On the other hand, when a car full of intoxicated youths crashes on the freeway and several are killed and several are severely injured, the possibility that all should have been saved given proper medical management is almost never raised. In this case, no one hears of any problems with medical management; almost no one expects that individuals involved in such an event should have survived; and it often appears that almost no one cares.

HOSPITALS

The Hospital Council of Southern California and individual hospital administrators have long apparently believed that the problem of trauma care was being adequately addressed by members of their respective medical staffs. Faith in the system combined with an abiding fear that evolution of a trauma system might very well reduce patient loads or even eliminate individual hospitals from the system has resulted in a lack of enthusiasm for addressing the problem. When faced with the necessity to cope with numerous unscheduled surgeries, the need for a system of emergency department management, operating suite availability, intensive care unit bed capacity, and adequate support equipment and personnel, many hospitals have simply chosen to avoid the issue.

Certainly trauma has the reputation of disrupting orderly hospital administration, precluding elective surgery, and potentially filling beds with undesirables who cannot or will not pay the cost of their care. These considerations and many more have led to a quite reasonable general lack of enthusiasm for reaching a solution to the problem.

PHYSICIANS

Emergency Physicians

While one might expect that both the American College of Emergency Physicians and individual emergency doctors would be wildly enthusiastic about improving trauma care, it is not clear that this is the case. Some individual emergency physicians have voiced strenuous opposition to any change in the status quo based on the perception that trauma centers would be run by surgeons, excluding the emergency medical community from participation.

Another widely held view among emergency physicians is that mere addition of a "trauma system" component to the current "nonsystem" of emergency care will only increase cost and propagate chaos. Without a very basic reorganization of the entire system to include all components of emergency care, complete with an accepted administrative structure and leadership with control and enforcement power, no "band-aid" repair is worth the effort.

Surgeons

In my view, it has been a long-held misconception that any surgeon can do trauma surgery any time. Anyone evaluating, even superficially, the problem of trauma care will recognize that trauma surgery is a specialty in itself. Traumatologists, while currently few in number, can and should be trained. Such individuals familiar with the needs of the trauma patients can do much to improve care of trauma victims. The idea that any general or cardiothoracic surgeon can be called on to manage trauma is unreasonable at best.

The fact that trauma is unscheduled and hence interferes with the orderly practice of surgical medicine makes it difficult for even the trained and willing surgeon to be readily and consistently available. Given a ready and willing general surgeon, unless that physician has sufficient regular opportunity to resuscitate and manage trauma victims surgically, it is highly unlikely that outcomes will be optimized by his or her participation. The solution to all these problems lies in the creation of a system of care that provides for surgeons.

The Rest of the Medical Profession

Although it is impossible to know the perceptions and attitudes of the majority of physicians, one can safely say that there has been no outpouring of public participation by the medical profession in local or national attempts to rectify the problem of trauma care. As is generally the case, a very small number of dedicated and at times driven physicians find themselves saddled with responsibility for the solution of a problem about which they know little. Attempts to familiarize themselves with the problems, participate in public and political discussion, and bring to bear the necessary energy and activity required for a successful solution frequently leads to early burn-out, bruised elbows, and a willingness to escape into the privacy of one's own private medical domain. Lack of a widely recognized data base and minimal cooperation between representatives of various components of the emergency system make it difficult if not impossible to reach a solution.

NURSES

While the nursing profession has evolved tremendously over the past few years to become an integral and crucial element in the delivery of prehospital and emergency care, nurses remain underrepresented in movements involved in reaching a solution to the problem of trauma care. However, it is gratifying to note the rising swell of support and notable representation from individuals of both Emergency Department Nurses Association (EDNA) and the nursing profession in general.

PARAMEDIC PROVIDERS

The major providers of prehospital care in Los Angeles County are the fire departments of the cities that make up this geographical area. While those who lead these agencies clearly desire an orderly system of trauma care, they are justifiably wary of a system that threatens to break the back of an already thinly stretched prehospital care system. Lengthening transport times by bypassing hospitals to go to a "better hospital," although logical and supported by medical data, seems at best an additional burden on a system that is being taxed already.

The shrinking financial support for this system, the rising patient load, and increasing public expectation all come together in a fashion which guaranteed that public provider agencies will find it difficult to support added responsibilities enthusiastically, unless there is concomitant financial and medical support. Furthermore, providers and individual paramedics find themselves quite justifiably wary of complex field triage protocols, unclear lines of authority, and potentially increased medical-legal responsibilities. Without a willingness on the part of the community to address these issues financially and administratively, one could hardly expect the enthusiastic participation of provider agencies in any movement to alter the current system dramatically.

POLITICIANS

The fact that trauma care has become a public issue is obvious. Unfortunately, the introduction of this matter into the political arena, while absolutely necessary in order to reach a successful conclusion, at the same time, reemphasizes the absence of a central, authoritative, "buck stops here" agency or individual who has the power and authority and general support to orchestrate a solution to problems in emergency health care. The fact that the ongoing battle over who is in charge has not yet been solved protracts and enlarges a problem that is already difficult without the addition of political chaos.

The Los Angeles City Council, the Los Angeles City Fire Department, the Los Angeles County Board of Supervisors, the Los Angeles County Fire Department, the Los Angeles Emergency Medical Care Commission, Los Angeles County Medical Association, California Fire Chiefs Association, the Chief Administrative Officer of Los

Angeles County, and a host of other political individuals and agencies are all actively involved in expressing their perceptions of the problem and their recommendations for its solution. Even if one or more of these agencies were willing to accept the full responsibility, there is unwillingness on the part of the rest to allow that responsibility to be shifted to any one identifiable final authority.

Public funding, of necessity a consideration of the political agencies and individuals involved in this lengthy battle, is a rising problem. In a time when we need more money to meet ever-increasing numbers of trauma patient problems, less money is voted by the citizenry. Hard times are upon us, and I am afraid that quite often the general wisdom is, "We've done without it in good times, why do we need it in hard times?"

ACADEMIC CIRCLES

Again, it is difficult to speak in generalities. And again, there are notable exceptions to what is, in general, wide-spread apathy among the academic institutions that should be involved in this most important decision. The perceived need of individual departments to continue to work exclusively on projects of their own design has resulted in appallingly little participation by even those closest to the problem, the academic divisions and departments of emergency and surgical medicine. In general, trauma is not a part of any of the kingdoms in place or being built in the academic institutions of Los Angeles County. Most residency training programs include precious little trauma exposure as part of their organized teaching program. The push, on the other hand, is clearly in the main toward research, specialized surgical skills exclusive of trauma management, and the development and organization of hospital complexes to reflect those preferences. Without great pressure, it is extremely unlikely that any great changes will occur in this area. Research and data publication, certainly recognized major responsibilities of academic institutions, while improving significantly in the last 10 to 15 years, still reflect a decided underrepresentation of trauma-related research.

Public fundings for these institutions, while in the past quite adequate, has dwindled dramatically in the last few years, making it necessary for those involved in academic medicine to choose between a host of potential projects. Trauma has consistently come up the loser. Here again, it is imperative that the medical community, the political community, and all others to whom academic institutions answer make it clear to the leadership of these institutions that trauma care is a priority.

SUMMARY

Despite the multiple barriers noted, Los Angeles is in the process of developing a regional trauma plan. The most recent concept is that 10 to 14 Level I trauma centers will be designated and later evaluated. If the transport times prove to be excessive in certain regions, then consideration will be given for designation of a limited number of Level II facilities to meet the community's needs.

The hospital council continues to support the concept that any hospital that meets certain criteria should be designated as a trauma center. There is still a concern that when there are two or more highly competitive hospitals in a given region it will be politically expedient to designate more than one hospital. Unfortunately, the final decision in these life-or-death issues is likely to be made by politicians with a limited amount of medical input.

REFERENCES

1. Gill, W, Long, W. *Shock Trauma Manual.*

SUGGESTED READINGS

Foley, RW, Harris, LS, Pilcher, DB: Abdominal injuries in automobile accidents: Review of fatally injured patients. *J. Trauma* 17:611, 1977.

Fitts, WT, Lehr, HB, Bitner, RL, Spelman, JW: An analysis of 950 fatal injuries. *Surgery* 56:663, 1964.

Gertner, HR, Baker, SP, Rutherford, RB, Spitz, WU: Evaluation of the management of vehicular fatalities secondary to abdominal injury. *J. Trauma* 12:425, 1972.

20
INDEPENDENT PARTNERS: THE MEDIA AND MEDICINE
John Fried

On an excruciatingly slow news day in the fall of 1979, leafing through my copy of *Morbidity and Mortality Weekly Report*, I came across a small item detailing a decline in surgical wound infections in United States hospitals. Desperate for something to write about, I began calling infectious disease experts, surgeons, anyone who could talk on the subject of surgical wound infections and why their decline represented good news.

During this flurry of phone calls I reached a surgeon at one of Los Angeles County's large public hospitals. He listened to my question and then, with a tone of voice that clearly said he was suffering a fool, gave me his views on the subject. At the end of the discourse he paused and then, with only the slightest hint of sarcasm, asked: "Listen, why don't you do something that's really important? Why don't you write about the lousy emergency care indigents get in this county, about the way community hospitals do 'wallet biopsies' on people brought into their emergency rooms and if the 'biopsy' is negative, they dump them on county hospitals?"

That brief tip led myself and the newspaper to an eight-month study of emergency services in Los Angeles County. It was an effort that led to official investigations by the Los Angeles County Grand Jury, the Board of Supervisors, and by a reluctant Los Angeles County Department of Health Services. It was a journalistic push that brought about widespread changes in the emergency care provided indigents, to a reorganization of the county's 33-year-old Emergency Aid Program, and to a major impetus toward the establishment of a trauma care network in Los Angeles County. It was an effort that brought the newspaper a host of journalistic honors, including a nomination by the Pulitzer Board for its Meritorious Public Service Award, an award from Sigma Delta Chi, the Society of Professional Journalists, for Distinguished Public Service, and others.

The long investigation also engendered harsh criticism. Community hospitals, the Hospital Council of Southern California, and leaders of the Southern California Chapter of the American College of Emergency Physicians complained bitterly that we had unfairly smeared emergency services in Los Angeles, that we had sensationalized at the expense of hard-working professionals, that we had misled the public. That a medium-sized newspaper with a circulation of 140,000 tucked away in a corner of Los Angeles County could have such a massive impact, it was argued, was just one more example of the terrible and uncontrolled power of the press. Why the bitter reaction?

To a great extent the medical community's anger and bitterness were predictable. Everybody is offended when the media begins to ask questions. Politicians wrap themselves in the American flag when newspapers investigate their activities, minority leaders vest themselves in hair shirts when reporters begin to wonder if more poverty funds have found their way into office furnishings than into programs for the needy.

But there are added dimensions to the fury that erupts in the medical community when newspapers or television news programs begin to probe. Contributing to the reaction is a simple feeling of betrayal. Doctors, hospitals, and researchers (even more so than other people) like to be treated deferentially; they believe themselves beyond reproach because, as far as they are concerned, they have only one goal—the annihilation of disease and suffering.

For a long time we in the media acted accordingly. When Christian Barnard, Michael Debakey, Denton Cooley, and others were transplanting hearts, bypassing plugged coronary arteries, and using jets of carbon dioxide gas to ream out atherosclerotic vessels, the media was there, agog over 21st century procedures suddenly emerging in the 1960s. We were there to herald advances in treatment of cancer, in the treatment of arthritis, in the new insights into the workings of the immune system, the coming of the Computerized Axial Tomography (CAT) scanners and other ultrasophisticated pieces of machinery, the "miraculous" emergence of antidepressants, and the exciting development of new non-Freudian psychotherapies. The media's role as acolyte has been appreciated even more when journalists have gone out of their way to skewer the medical establishment's hateful enemies: Adelle Davis, Rodale Press, chiropractors, and other alleged peddlers of misleading or unproven nostrums.

Because more often than not the press eyes medicine with a worshipful eye, medical professionals are totally unprepared for those times when medical writers bring out their own scalpels. Perhaps even more important, physicians and other medical professionals react angrily to investigative efforts because they are convinced that the reporter is delving into areas he or she cannot possibly understand. A reporter analyzing the actions of politicians, ghetto leaders, or bureaucrats is, in the final analysis, a layman scrutinizing laymen. A congressman caught with a handout cannot dismiss a reporter's inquiries by calling into question the journalist's ability to cope with the finer subtleties of political science.

But the anger that wells up in physicians whose acitivites are under journalistic investigation is fed by the conviction that this layman—someone who at best may have no more than an advanced degree in journalism—has no right to question the judgment or professional actions of people who have had years of intensive and complex training in a highly specialized and difficult field.

The medical reporter, it is true, does not have an inalienable right to sweep through medicine's halls and question everything that is seen there. But there is a responsibility to be no less conscientious about questioning what goes on in the medical community than general assignment reporters are in delving into the machinations of the local city hall.

Like other journalists the medical reporter needs only to answer three basic questions:

- What assurance is there that he or she is getting the best information possible?
- What assurance is there that he or she is getting all the necessary information?
- What asssurance is there that he or she is putting the proper interpretation on the gathered data?

Perhaps the best way to shed some light on the way these questions are answered is to examine some case studies: the *Press-Telegram's* investigations into the phenomenon known as patient dumping and the paper's study of emergency room deaths in Los Angeles County.

Our first break (before I started the investigation I asked Gerald Merrell, another highly experienced investigative reporter on the newspaper's staff, to work with me) came when the physician whom I had interviewed for the surgical wound infection story decided that he should be more than just another tipster to a newspaper. After several meetings he said were "let's get acquainted" talks, the physician—we'll call him Dr. Smith because he ultimately opted for anonymity—volunteered to make available raw data he had been gathering for a medical study of critically injured patients, their treatment, and prognosis.

His was a purely medical study, a project totally unrelated to the dumping phenomenon. But while the charts he had been collecting on hundreds of patients contained all the purely scientific information he needed for his own purposes, each folder also contained other interesting data: whether the patient had been brought directly to the county facility's emergency room or whether the patient had been transferred there from a community hospital; how long the patient, if the ambulance had first taken him or her to a community hospital emergency room, had been kept there before being transferred to the county; the extent of the patient's injuries; the name of the hospital from which he or she had been transferred; what treatment, if any, the patient had received at the first hospital; and, in many cases, whether or not there was an indication that the patient had sufficient funds or insurance to pay for treatment.

After we had taken almost two weeks to scrutinize the data for several hundred patients, several trends emerged.

- Many community hospitals in the area surrounding the county facility where Dr. Smith worked were routinely transferring scores of critically injured patients to the county.
- Very often these patients were being transferred even though they had received no definitive treatment. Patients with stab wounds, gunshot wounds, and patients with blunt and penetrating abdominal and chest trauma were being shuttled out of community hospitals without having had surgery and, very often, without having had the benefit of a surgical consultation.
- Very often these patients were kept in emergency rooms for hours on end (in some cases up to 10 to 13 hours) before being transferred to the county hospital for surgery or placement in an intensive care unit.
- Virtually without exception the patients being transferred were people who had no insurance, no visible means of support, and were black, Hispanic, very young or very old.

Did we have a story at this point? We thought not. The data we saw had not been analyzed. More importantly, it came only from one source. Although Dr. Smith was a ranking physician at his institution, although he had an impressive academic background and had served in several of the nation's finer medical institutions, we had no way of knowing if he had been as diligent as possible in collecting his facts, whether he had a bias we could not spot, whether he had spoon-fed us the information to manipulate us and achieve some obscure goal of his own.

We had to consider the possibility that the movement of critically injured patients from community hospitals to Dr. Smith's county facility, in a way we did not yet understand, constituted acceptable medical practice. Thus, we had to find out whether or not the same pattern of transfers was taking place in other parts of Los Angeles County, whether or not the rest of the 100 or so community hospitals in other parts of the county were also shuttling indigent patients to the county's three other publicly financed hospitals.

But we had a problem. We did not have sources in the other county hospitals. Even if we could dig some up it was highly unlikely that any one else had been collecting data as efficiently and ambitiously as Dr. Smith. Momentarily stumped, we decided to pursue another avenue, one that would at least give us some insight into the financial aspects of patient transfers.

By this time, of course, we knew that patient transfers were taking place in part because of Los Angeles County's Emergency Aid Program (EAP). Under the EAP the county had committed itself to paying for the transport of indigent accident victims from the site of the injury to the nearest community hospital and for the treatment accorded them there. Under the EAP we learned, community hospitals could transfer indigents to county facilities—but only under stringent conditions and only if the patients were deemed to be medically stable. Or so the theory behind EAP ran.

We reasoned that somewhere there had to be records of the bills that ambulance companies and community hospitals sent to the county for collection for sevices rendered to indigents. We found the office where those bills were handled—and in the process ran into a rich lode of information. Hospitals that had committed themselves to providing care for indigent patients, we found, could not submit bare-bone bills in order to obtain reimbursement. They had to submit detailed vouchers listing every medical procedure, every test, every medical supply used in treating the indigent patient. Moreover, every submission had to include a diagnosis for the patient, the time of arrival at the hospital, the time of discharge, and the place to which the patient had been discharged. In one central location, in other words, we had information for tens of thousands of transfer patients.

But how to make sense of all this? How to decide which of the 70-plus hospitals were treating indigents adequately and which were not? How to decide which patients had received good care and which had not?

Because we did not have the time or resources to analyze the performance of 70 individual hospitals and to scrutinize the care given thousands of men, women, and children, we decided to do what we called a "risks of the system" study. In other words, we decided that the guiding philosophical question we would try to answer would be: If you were critically injured, what was likely to happen to you if you were indigent and, as a result, funneled into the system Los Angeles County had established to provide your care?

To carry out this decision we chose, at random, 100 transfer cases. Three prominent physicians agreed to examine our data:

- A prominent neurosurgeon who had had broad experience in county facilities
- A specialist in emergency medicine who doubled as an academic, and who, like Dr. Smith, had also been conducting a very limited study of the care given critically injured indigents
- Dr. Smith

Each doctor looked at the data independently and gave us an opinion without consulting the other experts involved. We then tallied the opinions. When the counting was over, we found that the experts had agreed on the following.

- Between 10 and 30 percent of the patients had received questionable medical treatment in the facilities to which they were first taken. That is, efforts to treat or to stabilize the patient's problem before transfer had been minimal, if not nonexistent.
- A substantial number of patients who were hemorrhaging were being moved from private hospitals to county-operated facilites even before the extent of their bleeding was defined or, once defined, brought under control.
- Many victims with serious head injuries were moved although little or no attempt was made to assess the extent of their injuries or to determine if the ambulance ride would compound the effects of the injuries.
- Many of the victims with head injuries were moved even though they were in shock or in a coma, although no effort was made to guarantee their airways and although the ambulances in which

they were transferred were not staffed by a paramedic capable of rendering emergency care.
- Badly injured or seriously ill patients who should have been admitted quickly to intensive care units were first kept waiting, often for 4 to 12 hours, in emergency rooms before arrangements were made to shunt them to a county hospital.

After several months of work, then, we had what we believed was an accurate picture of the way in which indigent patients were being treated. But was it a fair picture? Perhaps the experts we had consulted had been wrong in their analyses, perhaps they too had hidden agendas we could not spot.

To guard against that possibility, we sought to have our data reviewed by experts we had not chosen. We contacted the Los Angeles County Medical Association (LACMA), explained our project, and asked the association to provide an independent expert to assess the cases we had gathered. LACMA declined. We then asked the Hospital Council of Southern California, which by this time was well aware of what we were doing because we had already begun interviewing hospital administrators, to choose an emergency care expert who would go over our material. The Hospital Council, too, refused.

As a last resort—and well aware that it was not the best possible solution—we called the emergency room director of one of the hospitals that participated in the Emergency Aid Program. He agreed to look at our material. And much to our surprise in 96 percent of the cases he was in agreement with the other physicians we had consulted. About 70 percent of our sample of 100 patients, he said, had apparently received adequate care. Up to 30 percent, he said had been poorly treated.

Now, one other question had yet to be answered: Were community hospitals in Los Angeles County capable of dispensing life-saving care to critically injured men and women—even if these patients had the financial wherewithall to pay for their treatment?

With the help of Dr. John West, I designed a study that would examine the experiences of patients who had died in community hospital emergency rooms in the aftermath of serious injury. Three criteria were used to choose the patients to be included in the study. First, we would study only those deceased patients on whom the medical examiner had performed an autopsy and for whom a full autopsy record had been completed. Furthermore, since other similar studies had been criticized for relying only on autopsy data, we decided to look only at patients for whom full medical records were available. We could hope to do this because hospitals in Los Angeles are required to forward complete copies of the patient's inhospital medical record (including nursing notes, surgical notes, medical notes) to the medical examiner's office. Second, no patients would be included who had suffered central nervous system damage. Third, patients would only be included in the study if they had died after spending more than 30 minutes in the hospital. Because we had set these stringent criteria, I had to spend several weeks poring through medical examiner records to find a sufficient number of cases to analyze.

The effort was prolonged not because so few trauma patients died in community hospitals, but because hundreds of patients in recent years had not been subject to autopsies, because autopsy records were missing from many files, and because in many instances hospitals had failed to live up to the requirement that they ship records with the bodies. But when I had finally managed to put together 63 cases, the project went into its next stage: analysis by a panel of six experts in trauma surgery and emergency care.

These experts included: Dr. John West; Dr. Don Trunkey, Chief of Surgery at San Francisco General Hospital; Dr. William Shoemaker, Chief of Acute Care at Harbor General-UCLA Medical Center Emergency Medicine Program; Dr. Robert Rothstein, Director of the Department of Emergency Medicine at Harbor General; and Dr. Richard Cales, a practicing emergency room physician in Orange County.

Each physician was asked to analyze independently the data available and to make one of three decisions: (1) whether the death was clearly preventable, (2) possibly preventable, or, (3) not preventable. Each man passed his findings on to me and I then correlated the results. According to the panel, 7 deaths had been clearly preventable, 30 deaths had been possibly preventable, and 26 deaths had not been preventable.

Other interesting facts emerged about those who could clearly have been saved or could possibly have been saved.

- 54 percent were between the ages of 16 and 36
- 57 percent died after working hours (between the hours of 5:30 P.M. and 7:00 A.M.)
- 71 percent of those who should have had surgery never made it to the operating room
- 58 percent died in hospitals with more than 250 beds

There was no doubt that many critically injured patients were being adequately—even heroically—treated in Los Angeles County community hospitals. At the same time, our studies confirmed suspicions that the critically injured person, rich or poor, was gambling, involuntarily so, on entering the emergency care system.

The following are the lessons to be learned from the media-medicine partnership.

- By and large, the reporter, not the source, has ultimate control of the information that will run in the story. Moreover, the interpretation will also be the reporter's. The best a physician or medical researcher can do is take the time, trouble, and pain to try to guarantee that the reporter has the facts right and that the proper conclusions have been drawn.
- The reporter's constant worry is that the physician or medical researcher could easily act manipulatively by feeding the reporter one-sided data, one-sided interpretations.
- Because the medical profession can hide its mistakes under the guise that it is protecting patient privacy, the reporter can never be sure of getting the whole story when he or she seeks to evaluate a patient care system.
- Along the same lines, because the most knowledgeable doctors or experts often are not willing to talk to the press, the reporter, again, cannot be sure of getting the whole story when researching a medical issue.
- Because many knowledgeable doctors refuse to talk to the press, they are virtually seeing to it that the reporter obtains an incomplete assessment of the story he or she is pursuing.

The responsible medical reporter is aware of the pitfalls and accepts them as part of the dues for the privilege of practicing the craft of journalism. Those dues are paid willingly, moreover, because the reporter knows full well that he or she cannot work alone.

A political writer can spend hours examining contributions to a politician's election campaign and pretty much decide whether or not there is evidence of corruption. But a medical reporter looking through medical reports and charts needs more than a handwriting expert to help decipher the scrawls and notations that often pass for medical records. The reporter needs help interpreting that data. He or she needs to consult physicians who have different fields of expertise; a neurosurgeon, obviously, will look at a trauma patient and see problems that someone who is an expert in abdominal and chest trauma will miss and vice versa. He or she needs to consult physicians who have opposing points of view. A considerable portion of medical care, after all, is still art and not a science; and is, therefore, subject to different interpretations.

(In going through the medical examiner's file during my trauma death study, I came across only one chart that contained information even a first-year medical writer could depend on. This was the record of a patient who had received what can only be termed abominable care in a local emergency room. And that was clear not just because it was obvious that care had not matched the patient's needs, but because the nurse who had been charged with keeping notes in the emergency room had the neatest, clearest handwriting I had ever seen anywhere. In fact, after reading page after page of her fastidious handwriting, I almost began to suspect that she was trying very hard to make sure that she was writing very, very legibly.)

Ultimately, of course, the medical reporter must ask this question: How can the reporter, the readers, and, of course, the professionals who have been the subject of the inquisition be sure that the information that has been gathered, even if medically accurate, has been woven into a fair story?

Those of us who write for the lay press do not have to follow the same rules and regulations that govern health professionals writing for scientific journals. We do not have to subject our data to rigorous statistical analysis that the medical researcher uses to validate data.

But we can be sure that we are correct in our analysis of a situation if our studies coincide with those performed by people who are more expert in constructing and carrying out scientific studies. Thus, at the *Press-Telegram* we could be confident that the trauma study hit close to the truth because our statistics conformed fairly well to those elicited by other trauma studies conducted elsewhere by professional investigators interested in the problem.

For most stories, stringent statistical analysis is not possible. To justify printing these the reporter must be convinced that the documents to which he or she has access can be trusted—and perhaps more important—that the people giving information are credible. Time and experience teach the reporter the art of "diagnosing" accurately the validity of the sources for the story.

Furthermore, the reporter can also be fairly sure of being on the right track after obtaining indirect, but repeated, confirmation that he or she is pursuing a legitimate story. In the case of the dumping story we were not only convinced by critics of the Emergency Aid Program, we were convinced by hospital administrators who listed all the reasons why their hospitals could not cope with floods of indigent patients—all the time denying that they dumped patients. We were convinced by emergency room doctors who could list anecdote after anecdote about dumps and who assured us that at *their* facility such practices could not be countenanced. We were convinced by doctors who kept logs of inappropriate dumps in their desk drawers but would not release specific information to me. We were convinced by county officials who steadfastly denied that anything was wrong but could offer no proof that the system they administered was working well.

Finally, a story must be validated with the ultimate "litmus" test: the act of publication, the simple act of presenting the reporter's evidence to the general public. If a story stands up to the critiques that must ultimately come, it has proven itself not only accurate, but fair and true. Unlike the errant physician, the errant journalist cannot bury mistakes.

This does not mean that a reporter can concoct any story and then toss it out into the public arena to see if it can survive. Libel lawyers, many of whom most reporters would swear would like their papers to do nothing but cover charity balls, earn their considerable retainer fees by working hard to prevent gratuitous reporting. At times the system does fail, as it did at the Washington *Post*. But it does not fail often.

In fact, the danger is not that a medical reporter and newspaper will fail to treat a story accurately and fairly, but that they will fail to be aggressive enough in their coverage of the medical community. The medical reporter who sits around the city desk waiting for a story to come, no matter how well that story is written, is not doing the job. If a journalist wants to serve the community properly, he or she should be out on the street looking for stories.

Aggressive reporting is particularly important in the coverage of medicine. All too often, doctors, health researchers, and other medical specialists will devote an inordinate amount of time and energy debating crucial medical issues in their own journals, in their educational meetings or societal conventions. But these same people will do little or nothing to air these very same issues in public, out in the open, when the people who are most directly affected by changes in the delivery of health care—current and future patients—can participate in the discussion and, ultimately, in the decisions that follow.

The aggressive medical reporting that brings medical issues to public light, it is true, can be alarming, annoying, and even disruptive. It can marshall public opinion, bring pressure on physicians, and can even disrupt the smooth workings of the medical community. But, it might be argued that these things might not happen if the medical community were more open with the public. If that were the case, the medical journalist and the people who read his or her stories would be part of the process by which the medical community makes its decisions and allocates resources.

But as long as this does not happen, the medical journalist's first allegiance will be not to the medical community, but to the readers to make sure that they are fully informed, that matters that touch their lives and affect their well-being are held up for scrutiny. The physician who feels a measure of social responsibility can only applaud the process, and, if he or she is truly committed to the community's well-being, participate in it.

EPILOGUE
John G. West, M.D.

Trauma, the neglected killer, is the leading cause of death for Americans aged 1 through 37, and the third leading cause of death overall. The cost to this nation is over 83.5 billion dollars annually. Tragically, many young and otherwise healthy trauma victims are dying needlessly because of inadequate trauma care. The solution to this problem is the development of a comprehensive regional trauma system. Such systems must ensure rapid and efficient field resuscitation and transportation to designated trauma centers. The trauma centers must make a major commitment to trauma care and provide, at the minimum, an immediately available trauma team led by skilled trauma surgeons.

Although such a regional trauma system represents the logical use of community resources, implementation of such a system has not yet been accomplished in many regions of this country. Dr. Charles R. McElroy has clearly outlined the barriers to the development of a regional trauma system for Los Angeles County. He notes that, for the most part, the medical community is apathetic about the development of a regional trauma system. A small percentage of the medical community is threatened by such a system and has actually fought against the development of a regionalized trauma plan. He notes that the hospital council has fought strongly for the concept that any hospital that meets criteria should have the opportunity to be designated a trauma center. Finally, he notes that the politicians have been unwilling to grant authority to individuals or agencies to orchestrate a medically acceptable solution to the trauma problem.

Epilogue

Although each region in this country will have its own unique barriers to developing a trauma system, it appears that many of these major problems are similar. Orange County was able to develop a successful strategy to overcome these barriers. Our first step in this regard was to establish a data base that proved beyond a doubt that young and otherwise healthy trauma victims were dying needlessly with the current system of trauma care.

Once the medical community was convinced of the life-saving value of a regional system of trauma care, they were willing, for the most part, to give us their support. To obtain further support of the medical community, we found it essential to convince them that we were talking about only 3 percent of all trauma victims being sent to a trauma center. It was also essential to demonstrate that the system would be rigorously evaluated to avoid abuses. Finally, it was important to stress that any qualified physician could participate in the system if he or she so desired.

The problem in dealing with the hospital council proved to be difficult. In most urban areas, a satisfactory trauma plan requires that a few, but not all, well-qualified hospitals be designated as regional trauma centers. The hospital council, of course, believes that any hospital that meets a certain level of qualifications should be so designated. It is important to recognize that, in most cases, it will be impossible to change the hospital council's minds, and, therefore, it is essential not to waste valuable time in a losing battle.

The central point in establishing a regional trauma system is to have the plan accepted by the local or statewide political body. A careful strategy must be developed to get this plan accepted. The first step is to convince the political body that the trauma system is in need of major revision and to show conclusively that young and otherwise healthy trauma victims are dying needlessly with the current system of trauma care. A scientific study is not necessarily required. It is important to remember the value of a testimonial, both from the medical community and from individuals, who have experienced the personal and needless loss of a friend or relative. Additionally, media support, such as that outlined by John Fried, proved to be of enormous value in our attempt to convince the board of supervisors that Orange County was in need of a revised trauma system. And finally, it required dedicated leadership from the local medical community to negotiate the trauma plan through the various political hurdles until it was finally accepted.

Although the barriers to establishing a regional trauma system at times appear overwhelming, it is essential to avoid undue compromise. Unfortunately, many regions have been pressured into designation of hospitals with a minimal commitment as "trauma centers." Such a system will confuse and mislead the public, but more importantly, will fail to reach its life-saving potential. Once it has become clear that such a system has failed, one can anticipate that the critics will be among the first to step forward and say, "I told you so." To avoid this dilemma, it is certainly better to accept defeat than to allow the trauma plan to be compromised to the point where it will fail to reach its life-saving potential.

Fortunately, regions with established trauma systems have had the opportunity to evaluate their data. It is evident that regions with a major commitment to trauma care can provide data that documents the life-saving role of their trauma system. These data should provide a golden opportunity to impact profoundly the future development of regional trauma systems in this country. We must seize this opportunity to fight back against the number one killer of our youth—trauma.

INDEX

academic institutions, and trauma care, 158; accident evaluation, 138
accident prevention, 7
accident statistics, 8
accidents: helicopter, 109; motor vehicle, 7, 18, 86, 130
accountability, medical, 17
Achauer, B. M., 102
air evacuation during World War II, 122
air traffic controllers, 111
airway obstruction, 77, 79, 83; endotracheal tube, 84
alcohol intoxication, 99
ambulances: computer run sheet, 13; ground, 6
amputated part, cooling. 107
Antopol, M. R., 115
aorta: ruptured, 133; thoracic, 132
applicant hospitals: competition, 32; equipments, 30; financial considerations, 37; on-site survey, 30; score, 31–32
appropriate surgery, 133
Army, U.S.: combat support hospital, 117; disaster relief, 115; evacuation hospital, 117; general hospital, 118; medical corps, 117; medical department, 115; medical platoon, 116; medical research programs, 123; medical support units, 116; station hospital, 118
Army hospital patients, 115
Army medical corps hospitals, 117
aspiration, 83
Australian trauma care system, 9
autopsy, 129

autopsy method: age distribution, 144; data collection, 141; warning signs, 143
autopsy method of assessment, 136
autotransfusion, 83

Baltimore: fire department, 12; hospitals, 11
battalion, medical (*see* medical battalion)
blood pressure, 83
blood volume, 82
blunt injuries, 18
brain damage, 100
brain failure, 95
brainstem: decompression, 98; function, 98
burn center, 12

Cales, R. H., 17, 129, 141
California trauma care designation, 27
cardiac arrest: ischemic damage, 79; resuscitation, 6
cardiac injury, paramedic intervention, 79
cardiac patient: paramedic care, 77; as trauma patient, 78
cardiologist, 76
cardiovascular disease, 76
central nervous system: death, 141; injury, 79; lesions, 96
cerebral edema, 80
cerebral ischemia, 100
Champion, H., 87
chest, crush injuries, 132
Cleveland, H. C., 3, 14
clinical audit, 146

Colorado trauma care, 14–16
coma, 83; Glasgow coma scale, 87, 89–90; hypoglycemic, 98
combat hospitals: comparison, 120; nursing assets, 121; personnel assets, 121; physician assets, 121; shelters, 119; support, 117
combat medicine, 120
combat support hospital, 117
community hospitals: administrative commitment, 57; anesthesiologist, 57; emergency department, 55; 58; emergency physician, 57; financial considerations, 59; financial profile, 44–47; general surgeon, 57; medical staff, 14, 57; neurosurgeon, 57; newspaper investigation, 163–64; nontrauma emergency, 59; orthopedist, 57; patient discrimination, 163; patient mistreatment, 163; private, 56; reveiw, 58; size, 55; suburban, 56; task forces, 57; trauma care development, 56; as trauma center, 55–60; trauma center commitment, 58, 59; trauma patient load, 56
community needs, 5–10
community politics, 36
congestive heart failure, 99
Conn, A., 3, 11, 91, 108
consciousness, 97
coroner's records, 146
corticosteroids, 99 (see also dexamethasone)
craniocerebral trauma, 94
craniotomy, 96
curriculum of medical student, 154

data collection system, 42
death rate, calculation of, 144
deaths, trauma, 7; and arrival time, 137; causes of, 79–80; comparison, 133; head injury, 94; nonpreventable, 132; preventable, 132; prevention, 8; statistics, 131; survival, 131
dexamethasone, 99
dialysis, peritoneal, 96
disability, 8
disaster planning, regional, 64
Dracon, D., 3, 14
drunk driving, 7

education, 62
emergency care center, as trauma care center, 73
emergency medical technicians, 79
emergency physician, 63, 73; administrative control, 76; and cardiovascular disease, 76; duties, 75; patient management, 75; responsibilities, 74; and trauma care, 155
endotracheal intubation, 80
esophageal obturator airway, 83
evacuation hospital, 117
evaluation of trauma care, 141–51; clinical audit, 146; clinical method, 144
exsanguination, 79–80
extracerebral hematoma, 96
extremity trauma, 102

field care, 5, 74
field stabilization, 77
field triage methodology, 87, 89
Florida trauma care designation, 28
Fried, J., 160

Gazzaniga, A. B., 129
Glasgow coma scale, 87, 89–90
ground ambulances, 6
gunshot wounds, 12

head injury, 94; assessment, 99; CAT scanning, 99; circulation, 95; and corticosteroids, 99; of elderly patient, 100; emergency treatment, 95; management, 98; severity, 99; shock, 95; treating physician, 100; ventilation, 95
helicopter, military, 122

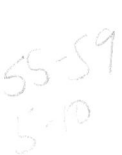

Index

helicopter accidents, 109
helicopter evacuation, 78
helicopter staff, 113
helicopter system: flight distance, 6; response time, 6
helicopter transport: communication, 111; and control towers, 111; cost, 109; cost-benefit ratio, 111; emergency landing zone, 110; hospital-based, 110; Maryland, 112; and medical personnel, 108; safety, 110; and state police, 112; urban areas, 110; and weather, 111
helipads, 110
hematoma: extracerebral, 96; intracerebral, 96; subdural, 99
hemorrhage: control, 132; exsanguinating, 77; operation, 134; and patient death, 134
hemorrhagic shock, 143
hospital chart, 146
hospital performance, newspaper investigation of, 165
hospital records, 143
hospitals: air transportable, 119; financial assessment, 39; operating room, 39; patient mix, 42; patient profile, 43; space, 40; staffing, 40
hospitals as trauma center, 27–36; commitment, 39; finances, 38, 39; growth, 38; image, 38; nondesignation, 52; training programs, 42; trauma load, 39; trauma profile, 43
hypovolemic patient, 81
hypoxia, 100

injured persons: care of, 5; transportation of, 15
injuries: blunt, 18; lethal, in field identification of, 86; mechanism of, 138; penetrating, 22
injury severity scoring, 22, 148
intensive care unit, 39; pediatric, 92; staff, 40

interhospital competition, 40
intracerebral hematoma, 96
intracranial bleeding, 80
intracranial pathology, 96
intracranial pressure, 80
intravenous fluid, 77
intravenous therapy, delay of, 82

Jacobs, L., 15
job description, 41
journalism, medical, 160–71
journalists, and physicians, 162

Korean War: helicopter evacuation, 122; injured soldiers, 5

lethal injuries, field identification of, 86
Lewis, F. R., 77
limb replantation, 102
Los Angeles: emergency room deaths, 162; emergency services, 160; trauma centers, 73; trauma deaths, 152–53; trauma system development, 159
Lowe, D., 8
lung laceration, 143

McElroy, C. R., 73
McSwain Dart catheter, 113
mannitol, 80, 98
Maryland: ambulances, 11; pediatric trauma center in, 91; shock trauma unit in, 113
mass casualties, military management of, 115–23
mechanism of injury, 138
media and medicine, 160 (see also journalists, and physicians)
medical accountability, 17
medical battalion: air ambulance platoon, 117; air assault division, 117; dental section, 117; mental health section, 117; optometry, 117; preventive medicine, 117
medical division, manpower of, 117
medical journalism, 160–71

medical platoon, 116; functions, 117
medical surgical beds, 39
mental status, 99; and alcohol intoxication, 99
Merrill, N., 108
microsurgery, 102; and physicians' assistant, 103; postoperative care, 103; rehabilitation, 103; therapy, 103
microsurgery laboratory, 104
microvascular surgeon, 103
military emergency, 116
mobile army surgical hospital (MASH), 117–18; air transportable, 119; physicians, 119, staff, 119
motor vehicle accidents, 7; blunt injuries, 18
motor vehicle deaths: age of victim, 142; data collection, 141; inhospital, 143; rate, 86, 130
multiple system trauma, 96

naloxone, 98
narcotic overdose, 98
National Guard, 115
Neel, S., 120
neurologic signs, 98
neurosurgeons, 94
neurosurgery, 94
newspaper, and medical community, 161
nontrauma emergency, 59
nurse coordinator, qualifications of, 41
nurses and trauma care, 156; pediatric, 92

operating microscope, 103
operating room supervisor, 40
ophthalmologist, 58
orthopedic surgeon, 6
otolaryngologist, 58

paramedics, 12, 77, 157; airway maintenance, 83; field assessment, 78; field care, 74; field treatment, 79; intravenous therapy, 82; response time, 148; role in trauma care, 16, 78; seminars for, 12; and trauma surgeon, 13
paramedic skills: clinical value, 78; complications, 78; effectiveness, 78; limitation of, 77
patient evaluation, 139
patients, hemorrhaging, hospital transfer of, 165
patients, trauma: airway obstruction, 78; death of, 79, 136–37; field care, 77; financial resources, 12, 42; head injuries, 80; helicopter transport, 108; hospital stay, 38; hypotensive, 83, 138; hypovolemic patient, 81; interhospital transfer, intraabdominal injury, 138; intrathoracic injury, 138; mechanism of injury, 138; neurological evaluation, 97; neurologically injured, 94; neurological management, 94; parameters, 51; pediatric (*see* pediatric patients); physiological condition, 78; prehospital identification, 12, 86; severed limb, 102; statistics, 9; transportation, 11; transport time, 81
patient transfer, financial aspects, 164
pediatric intensive care unit, 92
pediatric nurses, 92
pediatric patients, 89; drug dosage, 92
pediatrics: head injuries, 92; patient management, 91; social work, 92; splenic injuries, 92
pediatric surgeon, 91
pediatric trauma, 91
pelvic fracture, 144
penetrating injuries, 22
pericardiocentesis, 148
peritoneal dialysis, 96

Index

physician reviewer, 146–47
physicians, investigations of, 162
Pitts, L. H., 94
pneumatic antishock garment, 83
pneumothorax, 83
population density, 8
postoperative care, 7
prehospital care, 6, 78; evaluation, 23; medical control, 63; paramedic role, 77–85; rural, 14; and trauma surgeon, 74
prehospital deaths, 137
prehospital record, 146
prehospital resuscitation, delay of, 148
premature babies, 113
protective devices, 100
public education, 42
public funding, 158

regional disaster planning, 64
regional trauma system: analysis, 141–51; evaluation, 137, 144; and patient survival, 136, 173; statistics, 130–31; success, 129; and trauma deaths, 130–31; trauma survival, 131
rehabilitation, 7, 22; cost, 22
renal failure, 144
replantation center, 103; advantages of, 105; case load, 104; disadvantages, 106; laboratory, 104; location, 104; operating microscope, 103; patient travel, 106; postoperative care, 103; regionalization, 105; surgeon, 103; survey, 104
replantation surgery, 63
reporting, medical, 160–71; aggressive, 170; and physician, 168–69
respiratory distress, 89
respiratory failure, 83
resuscitation area, 39
rural communities: ambulance service, 14; hospitals, 14
rural trauma system, 14–16;
ambulance service, 14; finances, 14; interhospital transfer, 15; personnel, 14; and physician, 15; prehospital care, 15; training programs, 15; transport system, 16

seat belts, 22
sepsis, 80
shelters, expandable, 120
shock, 6, 95
shock trauma unit, 12
Simone, B., 86
spinal cord injuries, 12, 113
spleen, ruptured, 142
stab wounds, 22
state police helicopter system, 112
station hospital, 118
subdural hematoma, 99
surgeons and trauma care, 73, 155; responsibilities, 74
surgery, trauma, 74, 155; appropriate, 133
surgical beds, 39
surgical medicine, 156
surgical resident, 63
surgical wound infection, 160

Thompson, C. T., 3, 55
thoracic aorta, 132
thoracotomy, 132
tracheal intubation, 77
traning program, 42
trauma: communication channel, 13; complications of, 132; pathology of, 22; prehospital care, 6, 78; severe, 75; and surgical medicine, 156
trauma admission, 40
trauma care: communication, 75; deficiencies, 138, 152; efficiency, 6; evaluation, 17; improvement of, 5, 153; integration of, 6; medical accountability, 17; medical audit, 17–26; obstructions, 152–159; pediatric, 12; and physicians, attitude of, 154; political aspects,

157; poor planning, 152; problems, 17, 153–54; quality, 17, 144; recommendations for, 18; regionalization, 3, 5, 125, 129; requirements, 17; rural, 11, 14–16; success, 12; time, 77; urban system, 11
trauma center designation, 11, 27–36; applicant hospitals, 29–30, 32; community politics, 36; competition, 32; designating authority, 27; financial considerations, 37; interhospital competition, 40; medical considerations, 27; on-site survey, 30; proposals, 29; scoring system, 31; selection committee, 29; selection process, 28
trauma centers, 3; Baltimore, 11–13; cost effectiveness, 7; development, 36; economic considerations, 27; geography, 8; location, 8; patient financial profile, 45; political consideration, 12, 27; selection, criteria for, 33–35; staff, 9
trauma director, 41
trauma registry, 18–19; as audit tool, 24–25; and diagnostic procedures, 24; elements, 22; emergency department phase, 20; interhospital patient transfer, 23; operative care phase, 21; patient information, 19–21; patient transportation, 23; population description, 18; prehospital phase, 19
trauma research, 61
trauma score, 87–89
trauma survival, 131

trauma system development, 1–65; clinical needs, 67–123
trauma team: anesthesiologist, 6; neurosurgeon, 6: orthopedic surgeon, 6
trauma time, 39
traumatologist, 155
trauma victims, 3; age, 135; and nontrauma center, 138; saving, 129
triage criteria, 12, 138; low blood pressure, 12; refinement of, 150; unequal pupils, 12
Trunkey, D. D., 3, 61

University hospital, 61; commitment of, to trauma care, 65; economic issues, 64; emergency room staffing, 62; and government, 64; patient load, 62, 64; research staff, 62; staff, 62; staff training, 62; surgical department, 62; surgical resident, 63; surgical specialist, 63
urologist, 58

ventriculogram, 96
Vietnam conflict, 5; paramedic care, 78

war injuries, 5
warning signs, 142
Wernicke's encephalopathy, 98
West, J. G., 8, 129, 141, 172
West Germany, trauma care in, 6
Wheeler, D. A., 86
Williams, M., 3, 27, 37
World War II, air evacuation during, 122